Brian Duscha Publishing
5 Sabre Ct
Durham, North Carolina, 27713

Copyright © 2015

All rights reserved. This book may not be reproduced in whole or in part, stored in a retrieval system, or transmitted in any form or by any means – electronic, mechanical, or other without written permission from the publisher. For information about permission to reproduce any part of this book, write to:

Permissions, Brian Duscha Publishing
5 Sabre Ct
Durham, North Carolina 27713

Printed in the United States of America
Book design, editing and illustrations by Tom Dunne

FORWARD

Peripheral Artery Disease (PAD) is a major medical problem that results from atherosclerosis or "hardening of the arteries." Despite PAD being a manifestation of atherosclerosis, just like heart disease and stroke, it is a disease which for too many years has been under-recognized, under-appreciated, and far worse, under-diagnosed. This holds true for both within the medical as well as the lay community. There are a number of reasons for this. First, all too often the signs and symptoms of PAD have been ascribed to the "indignities of aging" and therefore not raised as a complaint by patients and not asked by health care providers. Second, oftentimes the pain caused by PAD can be very similar to and/or can overlap the symptoms caused by other conditions, such as diabetes mellitus or arthritis. Third, recent studies have provided much information regarding success rates of different treatment options for PAD. It is important that individuals with PAD, as well as family members and care givers of those with PAD, learn about and better understand PAD. This book is a valuable tool for health education. The book is comprehensive, well-written, and appropriately broken down to be understood by those with or without extensive medical expertise. The authors have carefully gone through and critically reviewed important scientific literature in the field of PAD. This book promises to become one of the best and widely read resources on this important subject.

Brian H. Annex, MD
Professor of Medicine
Chief, Division of Cardiovascular Medicine
University of Virginia School of Medicine

PURPOSE

The purpose of this book is to give accurate information about Peripheral Artery Disease (PAD) so that patients with PAD can have more informed dialogue with their care givers, family members and especially their doctors. By better understanding the information your doctors are telling you, and having read about potential treatment options, a patient can have more meaningful communication and shared decision making with their doctors. The information is intended to focus on leg pain that is brought on by walking and relieved with rest (intermittent claudication). This book will not go into great detail on the more severe form of PAD called critical limb ischemia. The motivation for this book comes from hearing patients with PAD continue to say there is not a book written on PAD that answers their questions or describes all areas of the disease. This book is a result of listening to the concerns and questions of PAD patients and trying to provide information and answers. The goal is to help you understand why people get PAD, how it is diagnosed, what your treatment options are and to help you prevent worsening of the disease. A reader friendly approach has been taken by trying to keep the concepts as simple as possible. However, some areas of this book (chapters 10 and 11) do go into greater detail. The intent is to empower you with knowledge, thereby giving you the necessary tools to create an optimal treatment strategy with your doctor. Hopefully, information gained from the book will arm readers with enough knowledge that they can understand their doctor and their treatment better; and optimize self-care. As with most things in life, the more you know about a topic, the better equipped you are to manage it. Keep in mind treatment strategies are often based on individual circumstances and that new medication, procedures and devices are always evolving and changing. Doctors, like patients, are always learning knew information to better manage illness. Therefore, this book is intended for fundamental understanding and guidance. It is not a substitute for professional medical care and all decisions should be made together with your doctor.

Table of Contents

Page

1. Peripheral Artery Disease: Causes, Risk Factors and Progression...1

2. How is Peripheral Artery Disease Diagnosed?......................10

3. What to Ask Your Doctor and How to Develop a Treatment Plan...17

4. Treatment Strategies: Lifestyle Management of Smoking...23

5. Treatment Strategies: Lifestyle Management of Cholesterol..32

6. Treatment Strategies: Adding Exercise to Your Life................39

7. Treatment Strategies: Lifestyle Management of Hypertension, Weight and Diet ……………………………………52

8. Treatment Strategies: Medications to Consider......................61

9. The Relationship between Type 2 Diabetes and PAD………..69

10. What is a Revascularization?..80

11. Exercise or Surgical Intervention: Which is Better for you?...102

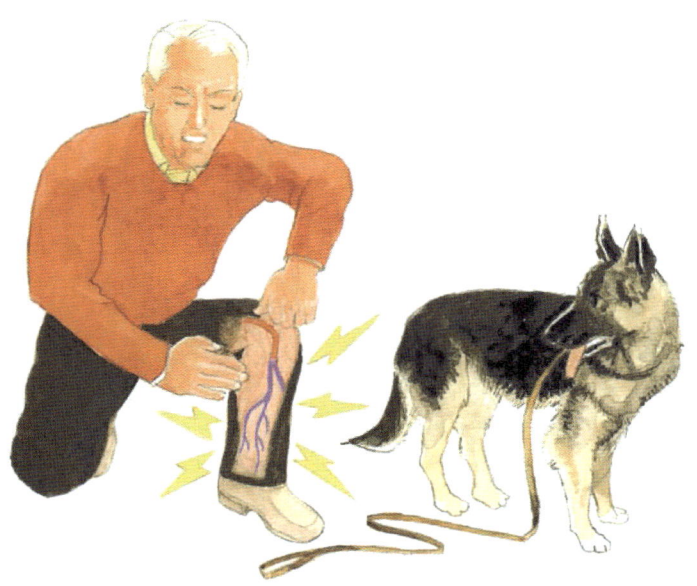

Chapter 1

Peripheral Artery Disease: Causes, Risk Factors and Progression

Do you get pain, cramping, tingling, or unusual fatigue or weakness in your legs that limits the distance you can walk before you get out of breath? Does this discomfort occur after the same amount of time or distance every time you walk? Is it more severe when you walk fast, up an incline, up steps or stairs? Does the pain get so bad that you have to sit down for a while until it goes away? These are classic symptoms of a condition called **intermittent claudication**. Do you have other risk factors for heart disease such as a smoking history, high cholesterol, high blood pressure, a family history of heart problems, or diabetes? If you answered yes to these questions you may have a condition called **peripheral artery disease** (PAD).

The prevalence of PAD is staggering. **Peripheral arterial disease, caused by atherosclerosis or blockages of blood vessels in your legs**, is becoming increasingly recognized as a significant public health burden [1,2]. Although long under-recognized and under-diagnosed in the medical community, and therefore viewed as less significant than coronary artery disease, PAD is now recognized to have a prevalence that is nearly equal to that of coronary artery disease [3]. One reason it is under-diagnosed is that people accept and think, as they get older, they should not be able to walk as far. Due to this mindset, it is

PAD affects 8 to 12 million people in the United States.

approximated that over half of people with intermittent claudication do not tell their doctor about their symptoms of leg pain. They simply believe their legs hurt because they are getting older and blame arthritis or being out of shape. One distinguishable difference is that arthritis pain does not go away after resting for several minutes. The Prevalence of PAD increases with age and affects approximately 12-20% of Americans 65 and older [1]. PAD affects men and women equally [4]. It is estimated that between 8 and 12 million Americans suffer from PAD. Many patients with PAD also have coronary artery disease and carotid disease (cerebral vascular disease). Therefore, if PAD is diagnosed, a full check-up for atherosclerosis in other parts of your body is recommended.

What Causes Peripheral Artery Disease?

The most common cause of PAD is atherosclerosis in the arteries providing blood to the lower extremities. However, there are other causes of PAD that include aneurysms (bulging/ballooning of an artery), fibromuscular dysplasia (abnormal growth within the wall of an artery), growth of cysts in an artery, inflammation of an artery (called arteritis) or congenital abnormalities. Although all of these do occur, these are far less common than atherosclerosis. Therefore, we will focus our attention on atherosclerosis as the main cause of PAD.

Atherosclerosis

The word atherosclerosis is derived from two Greek words, athero, meaning

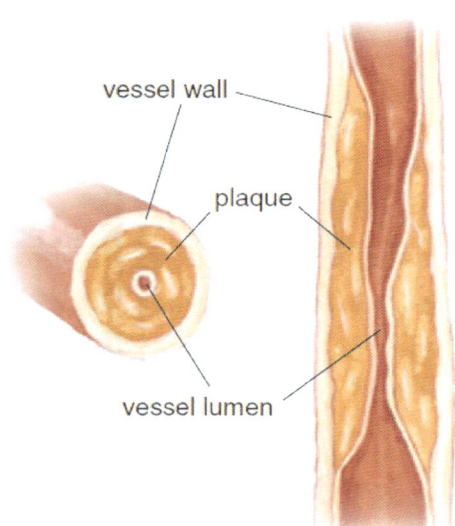

"paste" and sclerosis, meaning "hardening." Taken together, atherosclerosis is the process of plaque build-up on the inside of artery walls causing a narrowing or hardening that reduces blood flow (see left). The plaque is caused by a collection of cholesterol and fatty deposits in the inner lining of a blood vessel. These plaques may also become fragile and break off causing a blood clot. As we age, our arteries lose their elasticity and the walls begin to thicken. Although this is part of the natural aging process, genetic make-up and an unhealthy lifestyle increase the risk and likelihood of PAD. The disease process begins when the inner-most lining of an artery wall is damaged. This damage may be caused by a number of reasons, such as years of high blood pressure or smoking. A cascade of events then causes both an inflammatory response and the deposit of circulating fat from the blood to begin to accumulate in the damaged areas, thereby narrowing the artery and decreasing the amount of blood that can flow downstream into the muscles. This reduced blood flow results in less oxygen delivery, thereby causing claudication and potentially tissue damage.

Arterial or vascular disease is most commonly thought to be the result of atherosclerosis in the blood vessels supplying the heart. As arteries become more blocked, less blood is supplied to the heart. This lack of blood supply causes chest pain (angina) and heart attacks. It is important to recognize that atherosclerosis is a systemic disease, meaning it can occur in many parts of the body other than the heart. The word "peripheral" literally means outside of a designated boundary. In this case, it relates to the leg, which is peripheral to the heart. Atherosclerosis can also occur in other parts of the body such as the carotid arteries in the neck supplying blood to the brain or renal arteries supplying blood to the kidneys. This book will focus on blockages in the legs. Instead of developing blockages in the arteries of the heart, individuals with PAD develop blockages in the arteries of the leg. Similar to having chest pain (angina) patients with PAD get pain in their buttock, thigh or calf that is brought on by physical activity like walking. As described earlier, this **pain is called intermittent claudication**. The term intermittent means that the pain is not constant; the pain occurs with increased activity and goes away with rest. The term claudication comes from the Latin word claudicare, meaning "to limp." When muscles do not receive enough blood, lactate build up triggers sensory nerves to cause the feeling of pain. Simply put, the supply of blood cannot meet the muscle's demand so your leg hurts. This pain is usually relieved with a few minutes of rest. This can limit a person's ability to perform activities of daily living (e.g. walking to your car in a parking lot or working in the yard), or even impair someone's ability to have a job that requires standing or walking distances. In more severe cases, known as critical limb ischemia, PAD can lead to pain at rest, gangrene or tissue death, and even amputation of the leg or foot in some cases. The location of the claudication pain often can identify which artery is

Common Blocked Arteries in Relation to Claudication

Blocked Artery	Location of pain
Aorta or iliac artery	Buttock, hip or thigh
Common femoral or aorto-iliac artery	Thigh or calf
Popliteal artery	Calf, ankle or foot
Superficial femoral artery	Upper 1/3 of Calf
Superficial femoral or Popliteal artery	Lower 2/3 of Calf
Tibial or peroneal artery	Foot

blocked. The most common locations for PAD are the iliac artery, femoral artery, popliteal artery and tibial arteries. Depending on where the blockage is, claudication can occur in the buttock, hip, thigh, calf or foot. The location of the pain usually occurs at a place in your leg that is "downstream" or below the area where the blockage is located. Pain higher up on your thigh, hip or buttock indicates blockages in the aorta or iliac arteries. Pain lower in your calf or foot indicates femoral, tibial or popliteal artery blockages. The figure on page 3 shows where these arteries are in your body in relation to where pain usually occurs.

Risk Factors of PAD

There is an old saying, "Genetics loads the gun and lifestyle pulls the trigger." There is no question that some individuals are more susceptible to atherosclerosis than others simply because of inherited genes. Others seem to be protected in some way from illness. No one said it was fair. Science has made great advances in the last 20 years. But, unfortunately, scientists and physicians have not yet completely figured out how to identify those people who are going to get diseases and those who are protected from them. Until then, we all have to be conscious of what we can actively

Risk Factor	Increased Risk for PAD (percent)
Cigarette Smoking	200–500%
Diabetes	300–400%
High Blood Pressure	110–220%
High Cholesterol	120–140%

do to prevent and treat PAD. This means knowing the risk factors that cause and contribute to the progression of PAD; and learning how to manage these risk factors by practicing a healthy lifestyle and taking medication. Generally speaking, **the risk factors for PAD are identical to those of coronary artery disease**. This is because both diseases are caused by atherosclerosis. Because the underlying cause of PAD is atherosclerosis, PAD patients are also at risk for cardiovascular events such as a heart attack and stroke. Therefore, it is paramount to address all risk factors for heart disease if you have PAD. There are some risk factors, like age and genetics, that you have no control over. **Major risk factors that you have some control over include cigarette smoking, diabetes mellitus, hyperlipidemia (high cholesterol), hypertension (high blood pressure) and a sedentary lifestyle.** Each of these major risk factors will be discussed in greater detail in the chapters to follow. Other chemicals in the blood such as blood urea nitrogen (BUN), elevated levels of C-reactive protein and homocysteine are also important risk factors [5,6,7] that can be measured from a blood draw. It is important to know that once diagnosed with PAD, the disease cannot be cured or reversed. However, by aggressively reducing the risk factors and adhering to medicine, you can slow PAD progression and maximize your quality of life.

Progression of PAD

The most feared outcome after being diagnosed with PAD is that the disease will progress to critical limb ischemia and result in leg amputation. The good news is amputation is uncommon. In 1960, the estimated rate of amputation in patients with intermittent claudication was 12% over a 10 year time period [8]. Treatment now is much better. More recently, in a very famous on-going study which follows the health of individuals in Framingham, NY, only 1.6% of PAD patients needed an amputation after 8 years. Among patients with intermittent claudication, 16% will experience a worsening of their claudication symptoms, 7% will require lower-extremity bypass surgery, and fewer than 4% will need primary amputation. Approximately 1.4% of patients with intermittent claudication will progress to ischemic rest pain and/or gangrene. This rate is markedly higher among smokers and diabetics [9,10,11].

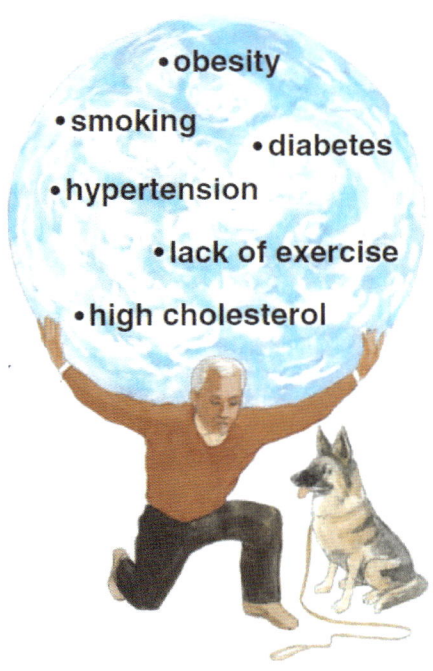

Risk Factor Burden for PAD is Similar to that of Atherosclerosis

The early stages of PAD often go unrecognized. In fact, 50-75% of people with PAD has no symptoms or mistakes the disease for something else such as general fatigue, arthritis, or accepts it as part of getting older. At rest or low levels of exertion, a patient with early PAD may not have any symptoms that something is wrong. As you start to exercise the muscle's demand for more blood and oxygen increases. Under normal conditions, more blood would be delivered by the arteries to meet this demand. However, if enough build-up of plaque has been accumulated in the artery supplying blood to the working muscles, oxygen rich blood flow is partially blocked and patients begin to perceive pain such as angina (chest pain) or leg pain (claudication). This pain is due to not enough blood and oxygen getting to the muscle doing the work. For example, at rest while watching TV, leg blood flow and leg oxygen demand is relatively low. Due to this low demand from the muscles, a PAD patient may not feel claudication pain until a blood vessel was 90% blocked. During light to moderate activities, it is not uncommon for an artery to become 50-70% blocked before claudication (pain) occurs. During walking, the blood flow demand can increase 25 times and oxygen demand 45 times above resting values [12]. A low supply of blood (caused by PAD), combined with a high demand of blood from the working muscles causes a supply-demand mismatch. This mismatch can cause claudication pain in a blood vessel blocked at only 50%. Over time, as the artery becomes more blocked, the classic symptoms of leg pain, cramping, cold extremities, and tingling become more noticeable with physical activity. Usually this pain comes on gradually as a person begins to walk and increases in severity until they have to sit down. Resting for 3 to 5 minutes will generally relieve the pain completely. It is very reproducible, meaning it happens about the same time every time (e.g. always after 5 minutes of walking). Walking fast or up hills will bring the pain on sooner. If left untreated, a complete blockage of an artery can occur, causing critical limb ischemia (CLI). This condition results in gangrene (tissue death), ulcers, nerve damage and eventually amputation. In very severe cases, patients may experience pain at rest while lying down or when their legs are elevated. Because of this some patients sleep in a chair or must periodically dangle their feet off the edge of a chair or bed to relieve the pain.

Increased Risk of Having PAD

Patients with PAD, but no history of heart disease, have the same cardiovascular death rates as patients with a prior history of a heart attack or stroke [13,14]. Therefore, the real danger for patients with leg pain and PAD is not the limitation of walking long distances or amputation, but for suffering a premature heart attack, stroke, or other cardiovascular complication. If you have diabetes, many believe your risk of suffering a heart attack is equal to someone who has already had a heart attack. The figure on the left illustrates that people with intermittent claudication have a greater chance of dying than healthy normal people without the disease. This is because people with PAD have a 4 times greater chance of suffering a fatal heart attack and a 2-3 times greater chance of having a stroke than those without, and emphasizes the need to aggressively reduce all risk factors for atherosclerosis. These threatening numbers make it very easy to understand why you have to pay attention to all risk factors of atherosclerosis.

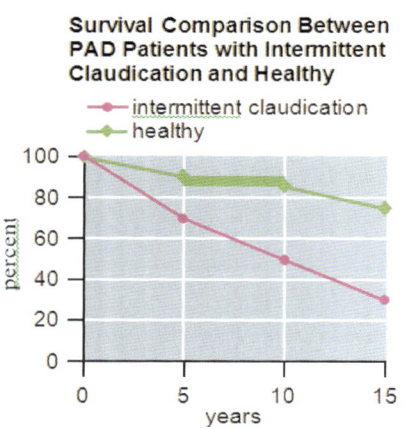

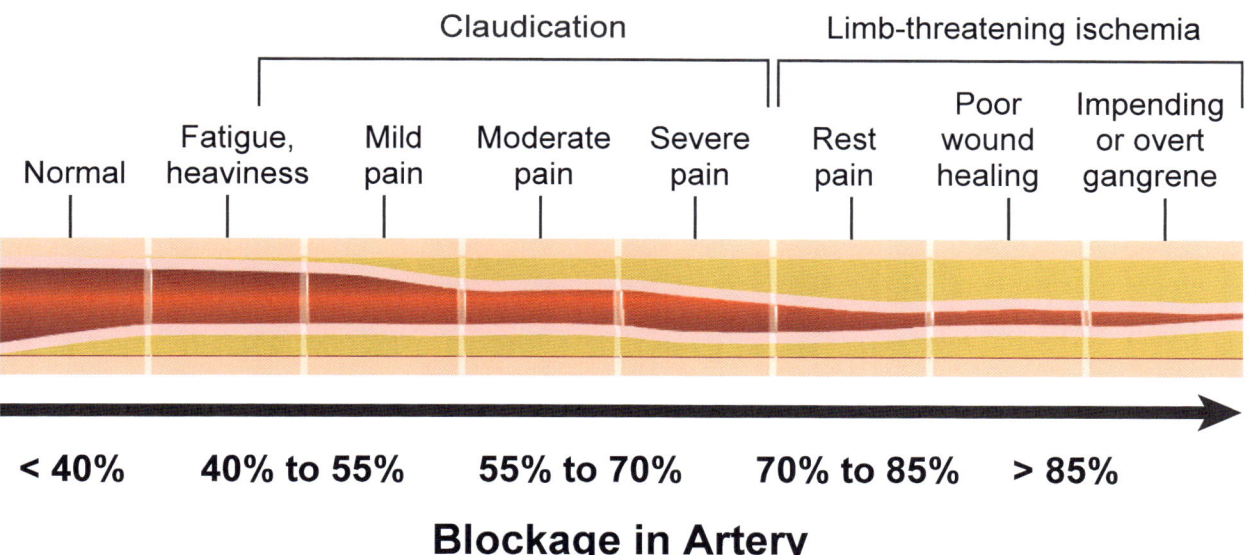

> **The most important thing to remember from this chapter:** Peripheral artery disease (PAD) is caused by atherosclerosis, or blockages to the vessels giving blood to your legs. This condition causes pain when you need an increased amount of blood and oxygen for activities such as walking distances or going up a hill. The pain in your leg is called claudication. The risk factors for PAD are the same risk factors for heart disease. The two most important risk factors for PAD are smoking and diabetes.

References

1) Heart disease and stroke statistics--2015 update: a report from the American Heart Association.
2) Fowkes FG. Peripheral vascular disease: a public health perspective. J Public Health Med. 1990; 12:152-9.
3) Kannel WB, McGee DL. Update on some epidemiologic features of intermittent claudication: the Framingham Study. J Am Geriatr Soc. 1985; 33:13-8.
4) Gerhard M, Baum P, Raby KE. Peripheral arterial-vascular disease in women: prevalence, prognosis, and treatment. Cardiology. 1995; 86:349-55.
5) Graham IM, Daly LE, Refsum HM et al. Plasma homocysteine as a risk factor for vascular disease. The European Concerted Action Project. JAMA. 1997;277:1775-1781.
6) Hiatt WR, Hoag S, Hamman RF. Effect of diagnostic criteria on the prevalence of peripheral arterial disease: the San Luis Valley Diabetes Study. Circulation. 1995; 91:1472-9.

7) McDermott MM, Lloyd-Jones DM. The role of biomarkers and genetics in peripheral arterial disease. J Am Coll Cardiol. 2009;54(14):1228-37.
8) Boyd AM. The natural course of arteriosclerosis of the lower extremities. Angiology. 1960, 11:10.
9) McDaniel MD, Cronenwett JL. Basic data related to the natural history of intermittent claudication. Ann Vasc Surg. 1989;3:273-277.
10) Hirsch A. Atlas of Heart Diseases: Vascular Disease. Edited by Eugene Braunwald (series editor), Mark A. Creager. ©2002 Current Medicine, Inc.
11) Weitz JI, Byrne J, Clagett GP, Farkouh ME, Porter JM, Sackett DL, Strandness DE Jr, Taylor LM. Diagnosis and treatment of chronic arterial insufficiency of the lower extremities: a critical review. Circulation. 1996; 94(11):3026-49.
12) Rådegran G, Blomstrand E, Saltin B. Peak muscle perfusion and oxygen uptake in humans: importance of precise estimates of muscle mass. J Appl Physiol. 1999; 87(6): 2375-2380.
13) CAPRIE Steering Committee. A randomised, blinded, trial of clopidogrel versus aspirin in patients at risk of ischaemic events (CAPRIE). Lancet. 1996;348:1329-1339.
14) Newman AB, Shemanski L, Manolio TA et al. Ankle-arm index as a predictor of cardiovascular disease and mortality in the Cardiovascular Health Study. The Cardiovascular Health Study Group. Arterioscler Thromb Vasc Biol. 1999;19:538-545.

Chapter 2
How is Peripheral Artery Disease Diagnosed?

Your doctor has a number of methods to check if you have PAD. These include: asking you specific questions about your symptoms and medical history, physical examination, measuring blood pressure and flow in your ankle, leg and arms, X-ray angiography, an exercise treadmill test, an ultrasound, or a magnetic resonance imaging test (MRI or CTA). The following is a brief description of each.

Medical History/Symptoms and Physical Examination

It is important to communicate to your doctor all information about your condition. Be honest with your doctor and do not think anything is "unimportant." The more he/she knows, the better their chances of treating you. Keep in mind the following things when talking with your doctor:

- When does the pain occur? Tell your doctor the activities you were doing when you felt it. Tell him/her how long it lasted and what area of your body was affected. Did it go away with rest? Was it in more than one area?

- How often does it happen? Every day or once a week? Has it been getting worse over time or was it an isolated incident? Does it happen only when you walk beyond a certain distance or up a hill?

- What exactly does it feel like? Does it come on suddenly or slowly progress? Is it more pain or more cramping/tight feeling? Does it burn, tingle or get numb?

- Have you had any changes in your life that may explain the pain such as a change in your job, a fall or recently started taking different medications?

> **It is a great help to your doctor if you bring a list of all current medications you are taking and the doses of each.**

Your doctor will likely ask if you or any family member has heart problems. If you smoke, or have ever smoked, let them know how many cigarettes and for how long (e.g. 1.5 packs per day for 8 years).

Important Signs and Symptoms of PAD Due to Decreased Circulation

- Reproducible pain or cramping when walking, pain goes away with a few minutes of rest
- Abnormal sounds (bruit) made by the blood going through an artery that can be heard by a stethoscope
- Weak or absent pulse on leg/toes at rest or especially immediately after exercise
- Abnormally cold feet/toes compared to other limb
- Numbness, burning or tingling in your legs or feet
- Unusual leg fatigue or "heavy legs" during physical activity
- Skin pallor (paleness) after elevating leg that does not go away after 30-60 seconds
- Difference in muscle size between calves
- Skin that is shiny, hairless, dry, scaly, or discolored
- Unhealthy brittle toenails
- Wounds, sores or ulcers that are not healing or bleeding
- A decreased sensation of pain in your toes*

* These symptoms are especially important if you have diabetes because it may indicate a more serious nerve condition known as neuropathy.

Physical Examination

Your doctor will likely listen, with a stethoscope, for abnormal sounds being made by blood flowing through your body. Blood going through a narrowed artery has a different sound than blood rushing through a normal artery. He/she will also listen to your lungs to rule out any potential pulmonary abnormalities. It is standard practice to measure your blood pressure because high blood pressure is a risk factor for both PAD and coronary artery disease. He/she will also touch your legs and ankles to feel for a pulse. Patients with PAD often do not have a strong pulse in their ankles. The skin temperature and color of your feet are also very important. Decreased blood flow can result in lower skin temperatures and abnormal skin color. Other potential characteristics of PAD include shiny, hairless skin or abnormal toenail health. Often, if only one of your legs has a blockage and the other has normal blood flow, there will be a distinct difference when comparing your two legs. The highlighted box on this page summarizes what your doctor may look for when examining your legs and feet.

Diagnostic Tests

Ankle-Brachial Index (ABI or Doppler Evaluation)

While up to 3 out of 4 patients do not report symptoms, there is a simple test to screen for PAD. **The most reliable, simplest, pain-free, least expensive test to screen for PAD is the ankle-brachial index (ABI) test** [1], which is the ratio of the systolic (top number in a blood pressure reading) blood pressure recorded at the ankle to the systolic blood pressure in the arm. This accurate test takes only 15-20 minutes to perform. While you are lying on your back, a technician will inflate a blood pressure cuff both on your arm and on your ankle and listen with a special probe, called a Doppler. This test is very easy, painless and accurate. **Readings of less than 0.90 are considered abnormal. An abnormal measurement means that an individual has a 90% chance of having PAD.** A lower number indicates more severe disease.

> **All patients with symptoms of claudication, known cardiovascular disease or multiple risk factors for atherosclerosis should have a baseline ABI test**

Many patients with abnormal ABI's do not have leg pain. This may be because the disease has developed at a slow rate, allowing a system of collateral blood vessels to grow around the blockage. Or, if a patient is very sedentary, they may not regularly exert themselves to the point that would cause insufficient blood flow and pain. However, generally speaking, less than 40% of patients with an ABI < 0.40 are able to walk more than 6 minutes [2]. The table at right lists ABI values and what they indicate. If your ABI is borderline or normal, but you still have leg pain when you walk, it is recommended that you get an ABI before and after exercise to see if the ABI reading drops after exercise. If the ABI drops below 0.90, or drops more than 20% this also indicates a diagnosis of PAD. Some individuals have arteries that are highly calcified due to diabetes or renal insufficiency and are difficult to compress causing artificially high blood pressure readings and ABI measurements of greater than 1.20. In these special cases, your doctor may want to use a more specific test called segmented pulse volume recordings. This test is also pain-free and requires

ABI Ratio	Indication
Less than 0.90	Abnormal
Between 0.80 and 0.90	Mild, possibly asymptomatic disease
Between 0.50 and 0.89	Moderate disease
Between 0.25 and 0.49	Usually severe, multilevel occlusive disease
Less than 0.25	Usually critical limb ischemia with rest pain and tissue damage

multiple pressure measurements on your leg and toes to assess your blood flow. Although an ABI is very accurate in detecting PAD, it does not tell your doctor exactly where your blockages may be.

X-Ray Angiography

This procedure involves putting dye into your leg artery while undergoing a lower extremity catheterization. An X-ray is then taken that allows your doctor to identify arteries that are blocked. This test is considered the gold standard in diagnosing PAD. The figure below shows a picture of a blocked artery by angiography before and after opening it by angioplasty.

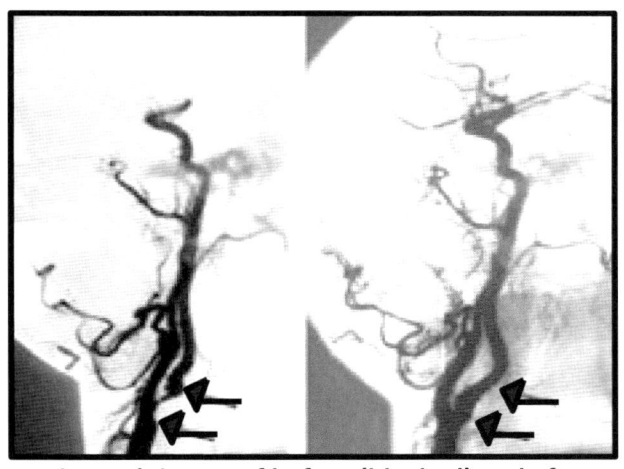
Angiograph image of before (blocked) and after (open) an intervention to open a blocked artery.

During this procedure you will be lying down on your back. Your thigh will be shaved and antiseptic will be applied around the area that the needle will be inserted. You will be awake for this procedure, but a medicine will be given to help you relax. A local anesthetic will be given to your leg to lessen the pain of the needle stick. As the dye is injected, you may experience a sensation of warmth or a strange taste in your mouth. This is normal, and should not cause concern. This procedure usually takes only 1 hour. Following the procedure you will be monitored for a time and usually able to go home on the same day. Although this is considered a very safe procedure, potential risks include: an allergic reaction to dye, kidney damage from the dye, excessive bruising or bleeding, or damage to the artery being studied.

Segmental Limb Pressure (SLP)

This simple non-invasive test involves putting multiple blood pressure cuffs at several different segments of your leg: the thigh, calf, ankle and toes. If you have a blockage in a blood vessel, the pressure will be lower below the point of the blockage. For example, if there is an occlusion in your mid-thigh (femoral artery) pressures below your knee (calf) will be lower. In contrast, the blood velocity will be higher below the occlusion. This is because the increase in velocity is necessary to compensate for low volume and pressure.

Segmental Plethysmography or Pulse Volume Recordings (PVR)

A "plethysgraph" is an instrument that detects and graphs changes in volume. Similar to the segmented systolic pressure test described above, blood pressure cuffs are placed at selected locations of your lower leg and connected to a plethysgraph. Each time your heart beats (cardiac cycle) the instrument measures the amplitude in a wave form. This is then compared to a normal wave (recorded in your arm) to determine if blockages are present in your leg. Usually, a difference of 20 mm or greater indicates a blockage. The combination of SLP and PVR is approximately 85%-95% accurate in diagnosing PAD.

Ultrasound (Duplex and Pulse Wave Imaging)

Ultrasound is a non-invasive method of obtaining images from inside the human body through the use of high frequency sound waves (2-10 MHz). Scanners emit and receive these reflected sound waves to create an image that can be displayed on a monitor. Each tissue in your body absorbs sound differently, and therefore the scanner can "draw" a 2-dimensional picture of your artery and the plaque inside of it. No X-ray is involved in ultrasound imaging. The image created shows the size, shape and amount of blockage inside your artery. A special type of ultrasound, called Doppler, is used to measure speed and movement of blood flow as well as the health of the blood vessel itself. This is called a Doppler Velocity Wave Form (DVWF). Blood flow to an area with atherosclerosis is different than blood flow in a healthy region of an artery. Therefore, your doctor can determine any blockages of blood flow and the amount of plaque build-up inside your artery in a specific area. Although no picture is created in a DVWF, many doctors consider it to be more accurate than an ultrasound.

Magnetic Resonance Imaging (MRI)

MRI has poorer resolution compared to angiography or CTA. An MRI can provide your doctor with a 3-dimensional image of the arteries in your body. This is a non-invasive way to look at not only the arteries in your legs, but also other places in your body like the kidney and neck. This method cannot be used if you have any metal in your body, have a pacemaker or other implanted devices, cannot tolerate contrast dye agents (renal failure) or are claustrophobic. There are no X-rays involved in this procedure.

Computed Tomography Angiography (CTA)

CTA displays images of your arteries better than MRI or ultrasound. Imaging takes place by X-rays passing through a rotating device at different angles. This allows a computer to assemble a 3-dimensional image of the arteries. Risks involved are radiation exposure, allergic reactions to the contrast iodine dye or kidney problems for patients with renal deficiencies or severe diabetes. CTA or MRI are usually indicated only when your doctor is considering a revascularization procedure (see chapters 10 and 11).

Exercise Treadmill Test

As you walk the demand for blood and oxygen in your legs increases. As described earlier, if your body cannot meet this increased demand, claudication results. Your physician may want you to walk on a treadmill to see if your legs begin to hurt. This is one of the primary diagnostic tests to determine physical limitations and disease severity. It may also be used to prescribe an exercise rehabilitation program or document your progress. Your doctor will be interested in: 1) how long it was until the pain started, 2) how long you could walk after the pain started, 3) the total distance and time you walked, and 4) the speed and elevation of the treadmill. Often, this test will also be used to test your heart while you are exercising by hooking you up to an ECG. A technician will monitor your heart on a screen and take your blood pressure during the test. The most widely accepted treadmill protocol (Gardner Protocol) is a constant 2.0 mph with an increase of 2% elevation every 2 minutes. **It is very important that you tell the person running the test IMMEDIATELY when your legs begin to hurt.** As stated earlier, ABI's may be done before and after you walk on the treadmill.

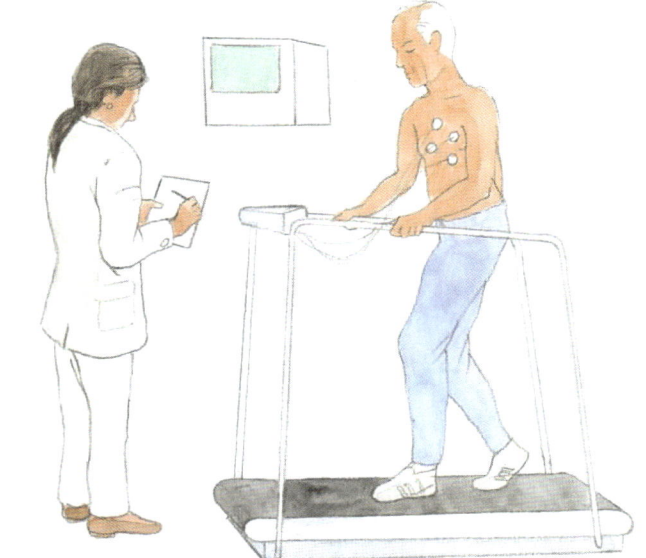

Summary of Diagnostic Testing

The type of test your doctor orders will likely depend on the reason for ordering it. If you are being screened for PAD for the first time or having a routine follow-up clinic visit, an ABI is most likely to be performed. If it is being used to identify the severity (area of blockage, percent blocked and length) of an occlusion in your artery to plan a surgery or angioplasty, then duplex scanning, MRI or angiography is the desirable test. If surgery is not immediately necessary, then simple SLP or PVR may be adequate. The latter can be used to document the progress of the disease and along with regular treadmill testing can evaluate the success of drug therapy, risk factor modifications and exercise training.

Blood Work

It is standard to draw blood for cholesterol levels and to rule out other severe illnesses such as kidney failure. Because we know elevated levels of LDL (bad cholesterol) or low levels of HDL (good cholesterol) contribute to blood vessel problems (atherosclerosis) it is important to measure these values. A complete blood count should be ordered to examine red blood cells (RBC), white blood cells (WBC), platelet count, hemoglobin, hematocrit (ratio of the volume of RBC to volume of whole blood) and blood glucose. If you are taking the anticoagulant medicine Coumadin (warfarin) and have a history of stroke, atrial fibrillation, pulmonary embolism or have heart valves; your doctor may also order a blood test to determine how your blood is clotting. This is called an INR (International Normalized Ratio) test. This measurement will help them determine how much medication to give you to prevent the formation of harmful blood clots.

The most important thing to remember from this chapter: **Do not ignore potential symptoms of PAD. If you are experiencing any symptoms of PAD, contact your doctor for an ABI test. If your ABI is less than 0.90, your doctor may order some additional testing to better define the blockage, such as segmental pressures and pulse volumes. If your doctor is considering either angioplasty or surgical bypass, you will likely also get an imaging test, such as ultrasound, angiography, CTA or MRI.**

References

1) Norgren L, Hiatt WR, Dormandy JA, Nehler MR, Harris KA, Fowkes FGR on behalf of the TASC II Working Group. Inter-Society Consensus for the Management of Peripheral Arterial Disease (TASC II). Eur J Vasc Endovasc Surg. 2007; 33(S1): S5-S75.
2) McDermott MM, Greenland P, Liu K. The ankle brachial index is associated with leg function and physical capacity: The walking and leg circulation study. Ann. of Intern. Med. 2002; 146:873
.

Chapter 3

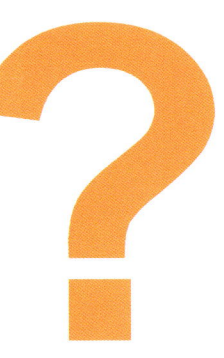

What to Ask Your Doctor and How to Develop a Treatment Plan

The goal of this book is to empower you with a general knowledge of peripheral artery disease. You can do this by reading this book and other educational material on PAD. However, because every person's condition is unique and different, it is always a good idea to ask your doctor specific questions regarding your personal case (1). First, make sure you understand how your doctor thinks you developed PAD. This may be because of a long history of behavioral factors such as smoking. Or, it could be the result of a combination of things such as untreated cholesterol, high blood pressure and inactivity. Or, it could be that you had an increased risk due to a family history of atherosclerosis. Knowing the likely reason for the cause will help you correct any problems you have control over. Below is a list of things you should consider when talking to your doctor:

- Ask your doctor if he/she can provide any guidelines or written information on diet and exercise. If you currently smoke, your doctor can direct you to a smoking cessation program or prescribe medicine to help you stop.
- Know the signs and symptoms of worsening PAD. And, know when you should call your doctor.
- If you are being treated by your family practice doctor, ask if he/she thinks it may be a good idea to see a specialist for PAD.
- Understand what medication you are taking, why you are taking it and the dose and what time to take them.
- Always ask your doctor when you should schedule a follow-up appointment.
- Although unpleasant, ask your doctor what the likely course is for your short and long term prognosis based on your specific case. Ask him/her what you can do to improve your health and prevent surgery.

17

PAD Patients can do the Following to Help Lower the Risk of PAD Progression or having other Cardiovascular Events:

- Before your next visit, tell your doctor you'd like an assessment of your fasting lipid profile (see Chapter 5 for details). You'll receive simple instructions before the test. If you need to lower your blood cholesterol, find out whether drug therapy or a low-saturated-fat diet or more complex treatment is warranted.
- During your visit, ask your doctor to suggest physical activity that you can do for 30–60 minutes, preferably daily, or at least three to four times per week.
- Ask what your ideal weight is, and if you exceed it by more than 20 percent, ask your doctor to prescribe a diet and exercise program. See chapter 7 for the body mass index (BMI) chart to determine your ideal weight.
- Have your blood pressure checked regularly. If you have high blood pressure, you may be put on medication. You'll also be told about other ways to reduce your blood pressure such as weight control, physical activity, moderate alcohol consumption and reducing sodium (salt) intake.
- Ask your doctor if you should take aspirin daily or another medication.
- If you smoke ask about counseling or nicotine replacement methods and other structured programs to help you quit.
- Always see your doctor regularly, follow instructions and ask questions.

Four Important Stages for Diagnosis and Treatment of PAD

Your team of doctors and specialists will go through a number of steps to diagnose and treat your PAD. Below is a list of 4 steps that are important in managing your PAD:

1) **Diagnosis.** This can be done either by your primary care physician or specialist (e.g. cardiologist). This includes a physical exam, ABI's, X-ray angiography, treadmill test and potentially other diagnostic testing (see Chapter 2).

2) **Consultation.** Your doctor will go over your test results and therapy options, along with their risks and benefits, and action items for you to consider based on the severity of your disease and level of risk. These will include medications, invasive procedures such as angioplasty or bypass surgery, and lifestyle management.

3) **Reduce Risk Factors and Modify Lifestyle.** Risk factors are all of the "bad things" that cause PAD. Based on your consultation visit, a strategic action plan to reduce your risk should be formalized [2]. This usually includes medicines to reduce your cholesterol, blood pressure and anti-platelets therapy (blood thinners). If you are currently smoking you will be told to stop, advised to start exercising three days a week, and eat a low fat diet. If you have diabetes it is important that it is controlled. At this time you may be referred to another specialist.

4) **Follow-up.** You should be regularly scheduled for follow-up visits to document your progress and trouble-shoot problems. These visits may include blood draws to determine if the medications are working (and not causing damage), if your cholesterol or blood glucose has changed a treadmill test to see if your claudication and exercise tolerance has improved, and a physical exam and ABI. This is the time to ask additional questions, have your medications changed and report what is and is not working for you. If you are seeing multiple doctors, it is a good idea to request a note to be sent to all involved so communication is not compromised.

Four Key Therapeutic Goals of PAD Should Include:

1) To reduce leg pain, improve your ability to walk, perform activities of daily living and remain independent. This allows you to enjoy a higher quality of life and remain both socially and occupationally active.

2) To prevent worsening of the diseased limb and avoid hospitalization, invasive procedures such as lower extremity bypass surgery or amputation.

3) To prevent or stabilize further atherosclerosis in other areas of the body like the heart or carotid arteries in the neck.

4) Educate you as to why you have acquired the disease, how to treat risk factors and incorporate lifestyle changes and when to recognize the need to see your doctor.

Unfortunately, PAD is not curable. Once you have been diagnosed with PAD, it is up to you to take command of your life and aggressively do everything possible to slow its progression. By doing this, you can maintain a good quality of life and prevent the need for additional surgery.

What Types of Doctors and Specialists Treat Peripheral Artery Disease?

There are a number of different types of doctors and specialists you may come across in treating your PAD. Although they all play specific roles, they also work as a team and overlap in your health care needs.

Primary Care/Family Medicine/Internal Medicine Physician

Until recently, many cases of PAD have gone undiagnosed. Initial diagnosis is usually made by a primary care physician (PCP) or a cardiologist. A primary care physician may recognize your symptoms or signs from a routine exam and suspect PAD. If PAD is suspected, he/she may choose to treat you themselves or send you to a vascular specialist (e.g. cardiologist).

Cardiologist and Radiologist

Cardiologists are considered "heart doctors," but because atherosclerosis is a systemic disease, meaning it can happen in other areas other than the heart like the legs, cardiologists treat PAD more frequently. Cardiologists are starting to look for PAD in all of their patients with heart disease because of the close relationship between the two conditions. It is becoming common practice for a cardiologist to perform an ABI on all heart disease patients as a precautionary screening tool. Cardiologists may also perform a catheterization or an angioplasty on your leg (see chapters 10 and 11). Vascular disease is now recognized as a sub-specialty and a board certification is now offered through the American Board of Vascular Medicine. A radiologist may also perform your catheterization or angioplasty.

Vascular Surgeon

If a surgery is required, such as bypass, a surgical specialist will perform this. It is advised to meet with your surgeon to go over all surgical options, risks and benefits and how to prepare for the surgery in addition to how to care for yourself immediately after. Ask your surgeon to explain the procedure, how long the operation usually takes, what you will feel like after it is over, what he/she hopes to accomplish, how it will benefit you and how long it will take to recover.

Other Specialists

Endocrinologist. If your cholesterol is abnormally high, an endocrinologist may meet with you to go over medications and other ways to lower your cholesterol. Another specialty of an endocrinologist is treating diabetes. If you have diabetes, you are at a higher risk for cardiovascular problems and may benefit from an endocrinologist's consult.

Exercise Physiologist. You may also benefit from an exercise physiologist to set-up an exercise program. Exercise physiologists specialize in exercise prescription across populations with special needs, like PAD, heart disease or diabetes. Exercise physiologists are trained in all aspects of wellness and therefore can give you recommendations and offer education on most aspects of risk factor reduction.

Nutritionist. Ask your doctor to recommend a nutritionist or registered dietician (RD) to assess your diet and consult you on a dietary therapy. Registered dietitians and nutritionists have expertise on food requirements for diseased populations. For example, they can help you meal plan to reduce fat or control diabetes, or how to time your meals around medications or exercise. They can help you lose weight and give hints on making food healthy without losing taste.

Physician Assistant (PA), Nurse or Nurse Practitioner (NP). These are physician extenders and often work in busy clinics or rural areas. They are often highly trained in a specific area, like vascular disease, and work together with your doctor. P.A.'s and N.P.'s often do your initial evaluation before the doctor sees you.

Anesthesiologist. If you are going to have a surgical procedure, such as bypass surgery, an anesthesiologist will discuss with you your options for anesthesia. These options will include general, epidural or spinal anesthesia.

> **The most important thing to remember from this chapter:** Understand why you have developed PAD and what your doctor's treatment strategy is for you. Make sure you know all of your risk factors and understand how you can manage them better to prevent the worsening of your PAD. Do not be afraid to ask questions! It may be a good idea to seek recommendations from additional health care professionals who specialize in specific risk factors. Talking with these experts gives you an opportunity to ask questions, better understand your condition and implement a thorough and detailed treatment plan.

References

1) Komaroff AL. Ask the doctor. My lower leg hurts when I walk. Could it be peripheral artery disease? Harv Health Lett. 2012; 37(8):2.
2) Marubito JM, D'Agostino RB, Silbershatz H, Wilson WF. Intermittent claudication: A risk profile from the Framingham Heart Study. Circulation 1997; 96:44-49.

Chapter 4
Treatment Strategies: Lifestyle Management of Smoking

Every 8 seconds a person dies of a tobacco related disease. **Smoking is the number one risk factor for PAD and is also a major contributor to worsening of disease.** PAD patients who also smoke are more limited by claudication than nonsmokers with PAD. It has been shown that smokers with PAD not only get leg pain earlier, but also do not tolerate stairs and walk less total distances before having to stop than non-smokers with PAD [1,2]. **This decreased ability to perform activities of daily living has been attributed to the fact that PAD patients who smoke also have lower blood flow to their calf muscles** [3]. It has been shown that smoking is a greater risk factor for PAD than it is for coronary artery disease [4]. The American Heart Association states that on average, smokers experience PAD symptoms 10 years earlier than non-smokers! Smokers have a 1.7 to 5.6 fold increase in the development of disease compared to non-smokers. It has been estimated that up to 90% of patients with PAD have a history of smoking [5]! **Smoking causes PAD progression, less successful surgical procedures, and 50% increase in death after surgical procedures.** In addition, PAD patients who continue to smoke have a greater occurrence of heart attack, stroke, amputation and death [6,7]. Even after taking into consideration all other risk factors, such as high cholesterol and diabetes, an incredible 75% of all PAD can be attributed to smoking [8,9].

The box on the following page lists several good reasons to stop smoking. There are over 4,000 chemicals in a single cigarette. The two most damaging of which are nicotine and carbon monoxide. Nicotine is absorbed by the body very quickly, reaching the brain within 10-20 seconds. Nicotine, besides being addictive, induces several unwanted effects on blood carrying arteries throughout the body. It stimulates the central nervous system by increasing the heart rate and blood pressure up to 20 beats per minute. Nicotine also constricts blood vessels leading to the heart needing more oxygen, which means it makes arteries all over the body become smaller making it harder for the heart to pump through the constricted arteries. And, it causes the body to release its stores of fat and cholesterol into the blood leading to a narrowing of the artery and atherosclerosis. The second deadly chemical found in cigarettes is carbon monoxide. Carbon monoxide from tobacco smoke literally poisons the oxygen carrying capacity of the blood. Carbon monoxide binds to hemoglobin in the blood 200 times greater than oxygen, thus allowing the blood to carry and deliver less oxygen. Heavy smokers may have the oxygen carrying power of their blood cut by as much as 15%. Carbon monoxide makes fat stick to artery walls. The result of smoking is that the heart must work harder than normal to overcome all of these detrimental effects. Cigarette smoking also increases risks of blood clots significantly. If the blood clots in an artery and blood can no longer get through, the tissue (muscle in your leg) that is supplied with blood has lost the source of its oxygen and nutrients. This cascade of events, as mentioned previously, causes leg pain (claudication) especially during periods of increased physical activity.

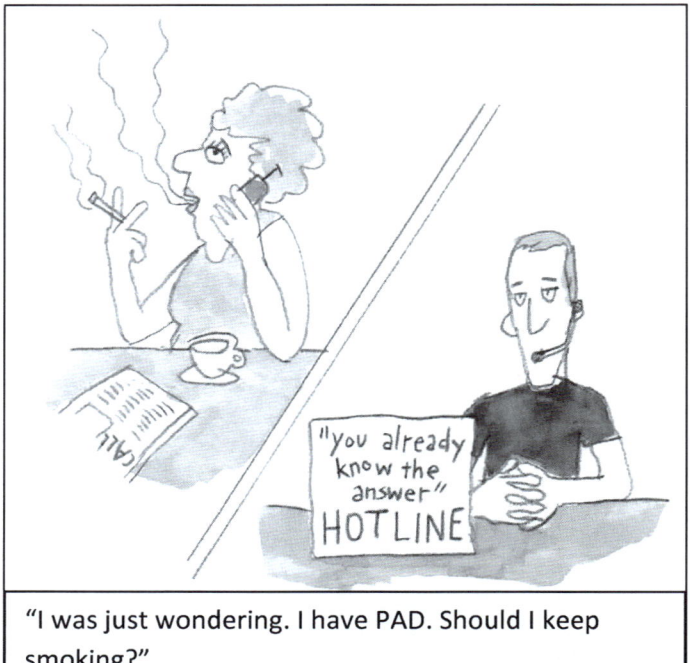

"I was just wondering. I have PAD. Should I keep smoking?"

Consider these 3 chemicals found in a cigarette:

Carbon monoxide – Also found in car exhaust fumes
Ammonia – Also found in floor cleaner
Arsenic – Also found in rat poison

In summary, smoking starves your body of oxygen, makes your heart work harder than necessary and, in combination with other risk factors like bad cholesterol and high blood pressure, causes damage to the inside of your artery walls, allowing plaque to deposit and accumulate. Cigarette smoking interferes with your blood vessel's structure and function, increases bad LDL cholesterol while decreasing good HDL cholesterol, increases triglycerides, causes blood platelets to stick to the blood vessel walls, negatively affects coagulation (clotting) and contributes to plaque instability---all of which promotes atherosclerosis and lead to both heart disease and PAD.

Benefits of Smoking Cessation

Short-Term	Long-Term
After 20 minutes: Blood pressure returns to that of last cigarette within 20 minute. Temperature of hands and feet increase to normal	**After 1 year:** Risk of coronary heart disease is reduced by 50% after 1 year.
After 8–24 hours: Carbon monoxide levels drop to normal. Your chance of a heart attack decreases.	**After 5 years:** Risk of stroke is similar to that of a nonsmoker.
After 1-7 days: Sense of smell and taste improve within days.	**After 10 years:** Chance of dying from lung cancer is half compared to those who continue to smoke.
After 1-9 months: Circulation improves	The risk of cancer of the mouth, throat, esophagus, bladder, kidney and pancreas are reduced.
Lung function improves up to 30% within 2 to 3 months.	**After 15 years:** The risk of coronary heart disease is that of a non-smoker.
Coughing, sinus congestion, fatigue, shortness of breath all improve	
Money is saved each month by not buying cigarettes.	
Patient enjoys increased self-esteem due to quitting smoking.	

Smoking Cessation
<u>A large amount of evidence shows that if you stop smoking, your prognosis will improve.</u> *Stopping for as little as 8 weeks causes improvements in blood viscosity and blood vessel function. Practically, <u>**PAD patients who smoke have approximately a 20% decrease in walking distance compared to former smokers**</u>* [10]. Furthermore, the time until leg pain occurs while walking and total distance someone can walk before stopping is improved for former smokers [11]. Last, the amount of time for the leg pain to go way after stopping to rest is also better for former vs current smokers. Those patients who stop smoking reduce their risk of amputation and have less rest pain than those who do not. Smoking cessation also improves long term survival in PAD. One study showed 82% of PAD patients who stopped smoking were alive after 10 years vs only 46% of those who continued to smoke [12]. The same

study showed that a heart attack occurred in 53% of those who continue to smoke vs only 11% who stopped. 46% of smokers died of a cardiac death, while only 6% of quitters had this fate. Simply stated, IF YOU ARE SMOKING, STOP!!!! Quitting is critical because continued smoking is associated with worsening symptoms, loss of walking ability, poor surgical outcomes, amputation, and death [13].

Recommendations

- Assess your tobacco use. Identify what stimulates you to smoke. Do you crave a cigarette after a meal, during stressful situations, boredom, etc.?

- If your spouse or other family members smoke, encourage them to quit as well. Avoid secondhand smoke.

- Find a substitute such as chewing gum or candy.

- **Less than 10% of people who try to stop smoking on their own are successful! GET HELP!** If you are unable to kick the habit by yourself, ask your physician to recommend a counseling program or drug therapy, including nicotine replacement. Currently, there are several drug options for smoking cessation. Any help you receive improves your long term ability to quit smoking.

- Consider the financial cost of your habit. **If a pack of cigarettes costs $5.51 (average cost in 2015) and you smoke 2 packs per day, you are spending $330.60 a month!!! Or, $3,967.20 a year!!!** Seriously, that's a lot of money. As motivation, treat yourself to something special with this saved money.

There are a number of recommended ways to quit smoking. These are listed at the end of the chapter. A brief description of each is offered below:

Nicotine Gum. Nicotine gum's therapeutic effect works by the release of nicotine by a special chewing technique. It requires the patient to chew slowly and periodically "pinched" between the cheek and gum in order to allow optimal release and absorption of the nicotine. This allows some nicotine into your system, but a far lower amount than smoking. The gum should be chewed at a rate of one piece per hour, up to 24 per day. One advantage of this method is that it fulfills the need of immediate nicotine cravings. Side effects include upset stomach, jaw fatigue and nausea. It is not recommended for those with gastric ulcers. This method has been shown to improve the likelihood of quitting smoking by 50-70%. Cost is $3.00 to $5.00 for 10 2-mg pieces and $4.00 to $5.00 for 10 4-mg pieces.

Nicotine Patch. A nicotine patch releases nicotine slowly and steadily through your skin over a period of approximately 16 hours. Dosing depends on body size and your level of nicotine dependence. After an initial amount is used for 8 weeks, the dose is then lowered. The application is simple (once a day), discreet and allows use for those with stomach problems. Potential side effects include insomnia, skin irritation, headache, dizziness and rapid heart rate. Do not share your patches with anyone else, and keep away from pets and children. Nicotine patches have been shown to improve someone's ability to stop smoking by 1.5 to 2 times. Cost is $2.00 to $4.00 per day.

Nasal Sprays. Nasal sprays provide the highest levels of nicotine and fastest delivery of nicotine replacement therapies. Patients are instructed to spray each nostril once. Each spray contains 0.5 mg of nicotine. Absorption is reached within 10-15 minutes. It is recommended to spray each nostril 1-2 times per hour to start, and lower from that point as tolerated. Possible adverse effects include nose and throat irritation, watery eyes, nausea, headache and dizziness. Studies show a person is twice as likely to stop smoking if nasal sprays are used compared to placebo. Cost is $5.00 to $6.00 for 12 doses.

Nicotine Inhaler. An inhaler works by releasing a vapor of 4 mg of nicotine that is then absorbed from the mouth. Each inhaler package includes a mouthpiece and 42 cartridges of nicotine. Patients initially use 6-16 cartridges a day (up to 12 weeks) to satisfy the craving for cigarettes. This is done approximately every 20 minutes. During the second stage (up to 12 weeks) patients are instructed to gradually decrease the number needed until you do not need them anymore. One advantage of this method is that it reproduces some of the hand to mouth rituals involved in smoking. The disadvantages are embarrassment of use, coughing, headache, mouth/ throat irritation, nausea and nasal/sinus inflammation. Cost is $10.00 to $12.00 for 10 cartridges.

Nicotine Sublingual Tablets or Lozenges. These tablets or lozenges should be sucked slowly and periodically "pinched" between the gum and cheek similar to nicotine gum. The tablets should not be chewed or swallowed. Lozenges or tablets come in either 2 mg or 4mg and need to be taken every 1-2 hours for up to 12 weeks. As all nicotine replacement therapies, the tablet should be gradually tapered as the need deceases. Side effects are similar to the use of nicotine gum.

Prescription Drugs. These include bupropion, clonidine, nortriptyline and varenicline (Chantix). Due to the seriousness of prescription medications, special circumstances for individuals and adverse effects on special populations, smokers trying to quit should consult both their physician and pharmacist prior to starting this method of smoking cessation.

Electronic Cigarettes. E-cigarettes have a battery source that allows you to inhale an aerosol that provides the sensation of smoking. E-cigarettes usually contain nicotine. However, e-cigarettes contain fewer toxic substances than regular cigarettes, and therefore may be less harmful than regular cigarettes. The balance between benefit and potential harm remains unknown for e-cigarettes. As of 2014, no major medical organization has recommended the use of e-cigarettes because there is not enough strong evidence that suggest e-cigarettes are better than the available prescribed medication or FDA approved products for smoking cessation.

Mark Twain said...

"It's easy to quit smoking. I've done it ten times."

Nicotine Replacement Therapies

Drug/dose	Duration	Availability	Form	Potential Adverse Effects
Nicotine gum; 2 mg gum up to 24 pieces per day for smokers of less than 24 cigarettes per day	Up to 12 weeks	Over the counter	Nicorette gum	Mouth soreness Upset stomach
Nicotine patch 21 mg/24 h 14 mg/24 h 7 mg/24 h 15 mg/16 h	Duration is dependent on dose, see your physician	Over the counter and by prescription	Nicoderm, Nicotrol, generics	Skin reaction Insomnia
Nicotine nasal spray 8 to 40 doses per day	3 to 6 months	Prescription only, see your physician	Nicotrol NS	Nasal irritation Dependency
Nicotine inhaler 6 to 16 cartridges per day	Up to 6 months	Prescription only, see your physician	Nicotrol inhaler	Mouth and throat irritation
Nicotine lozenge 2 mg or 4 mg Up to 20 dose per day	12 weeks	Over the counter	Sublingual tablet, lozenge	Mouth and throat irritation Heartburn/ indigestion
Sustained-release Bupropion hydrochloride; 150 mg every morning for 3 days, then 150 mg twice daily	7 to 12 weeks	Prescription only, see your physician	Zyban	Insomnia Dry mouth
Clonidine 0.15 mg/d to 0.75 mg/d	3 to 10 weeks	Prescription only, see your physician oral tablets or patch		Dry mouth Drowsiness Dizziness
Nortriptyline hydrochloride, 75 mg/d to 100 mg/d	12 weeks	Prescription only, see your physician		Sleepiness Dry mouth
Chantix Days 1-3: 0.5 mg once daily Days 4-7: 0.5 mg twice daily Day 8 – 12 weeks: 1 mg twice daily	12 weeks	Prescription only, see your physician		Nausea Headache Insomnia

> **The most important thing to remember from this chapter:** Smoking is the single biggest and most modifiable risk factor for PAD. Survival rates and symptoms of leg pain improve after smoking stops. Smoking cessation reduces the risk of amputation and improves surgical intervention outcomes. It is best to seek professional help if you are smoking, as few people are able to successfully quit on their own.

References

1) Gardner AW, Montgomery PS, Womack CJ, Killewich LA. Smoking history is related to free-living daily physical activity in claudicants. Med Sci Sports 1999; 31:980-986.
2) Gardner AW, Killewich L, Montgomery PS, Katzel LI. Response to exercise rehabilitation in smoking and non-smoking patients with intermittent claudication. J Vasc Surg. 2004; 39:531-538.
3) Gardner AW, Sieminski DJ, Killewich LA. The effect of cigarette smoking on free-living daily physical activity in older claudication patients. Angiology 1997; 48:947-955.
4) Price JF, Mowbray PI, Lee AJ, et al. Relationship between smoking and cardiovascular risk factors in the development of peripheral arterial disease and coronary artery disease: Edinburgh Artery Study. Eur Heart J. 1999; 20:344-353.
5) Faulkner KW, House AK, Castleden WM. The effect of cessation of smoking on the accumulative survival rates of patients with symptomatic peripheral vascular disease. Med J Aust. 1983; 1:217-219.

6) Hirsch AT, Treat-Jacobson D, Lando HA, Hatsukami DK. The role of tobacco cessation, anti-platelet and lipid lowering therapies in the treatment of peripheral arterial disease. Vasc Med. 1997; 2:243-251.

7) Smith I, Franks PJ, Greenhalgh RM, Poulter NR, Powell JT. The influence of smoking cessation and hypertriglyceridaaemia on the progression of peripheral arterial disease and the onset of critical ischemia. Eur J Vasc Endovasc Surg. 1996; 11:402-408.

8) Cole CW, Hill GB, Farzad E, et al. Cigarette smoking and peripheral arterial occlusive disease. Surg. 1993; 114:753-756.

9) Kannel WB and Shurtleff D. The Framingham Study. Cigarettes and the development of intermittent claudication. Geriatrics. 1973; 28:61-68.

10) Quick CR, Cotton LT. The measured effect of stopping smoking on intermittent claudication. Br J Surg. 1982; 69(Suppl):S24-S26).

11) Gardner AW. The effects of cigarette smoking on exercise capacity in patients with intermittent claudication. Vasc Med. 1996; 1:181-186.

12) Johnson T, Bergstrom R. Cessation of smoking in patients with intermittent claudication. Effects on the risks of peripheral vascular complications, myocardial infarctions, and mortality. Acta Med Scand. 1987; 221:253-260.

13) Anand S, Creager M. Peripheral arterial disease. Clinical Evidence. 2002; 8:82–94.

Chapter 5

Treatment Strategies: Lifestyle Management of Cholesterol

Cholesterol is necessary for your body to function properly. Your liver makes cholesterol to produce things like hormones, cell membranes and vitamin D. However, too much of the wrong kind of cholesterol in your blood can result in damage to artery walls. When your doctor talks about cholesterol, they are really talking about your "lipoprotein panel or lipid panel." Cholesterol (or lipids) is a waxy substance and therefore does not mix with blood. In order to transport this waxy substance, your liver attaches it to a protein molecule. That is where the term "lipoprotein" comes from.

Your lipid panel is identified by a blood draw and consists of total cholesterol, HDL (good cholesterol), LDL (bad cholesterol), and triglycerides. Because PAD is caused by atherosclerosis just like heart disease is, it is common for patients with PAD to have elevated LDL cholesterol levels and triglyceride levels and low HDL cholesterol levels. For this reason, it is very important to maintain optimal cholesterol values because **bad cholesterol (LDL) in your blood stream over time is deposited in your arteries and may cause further narrowing and leg pain. HDL is called "good cholesterol" because it actually takes the "bad cholesterol" out of your blood.**

As LDL cholesterol and triglycerides travel through your blood stream, it is drawn into cells to do work and is used for energy. The HDL's transport cholesterol back to the liver for disposal. However, when you eat too much cholesterol or your body makes too much cholesterol due to genetics, the bloodstream becomes concentrated with more LDL's than the body can use. This causes the excess particles to attach or stick to the inside of your arteries, forming the plaque that causes atherosclerosis. The following figure illustrates what happens when cholesterol is in and out of balance in your blood.

When everything is in balance...

Cholesterol is produced in the liver as very-low density lipoproteins (VLDL's) and circulates in the blood.

Some VLDL's go back to the liver.

Other VLDL's are carried back by HDL's.

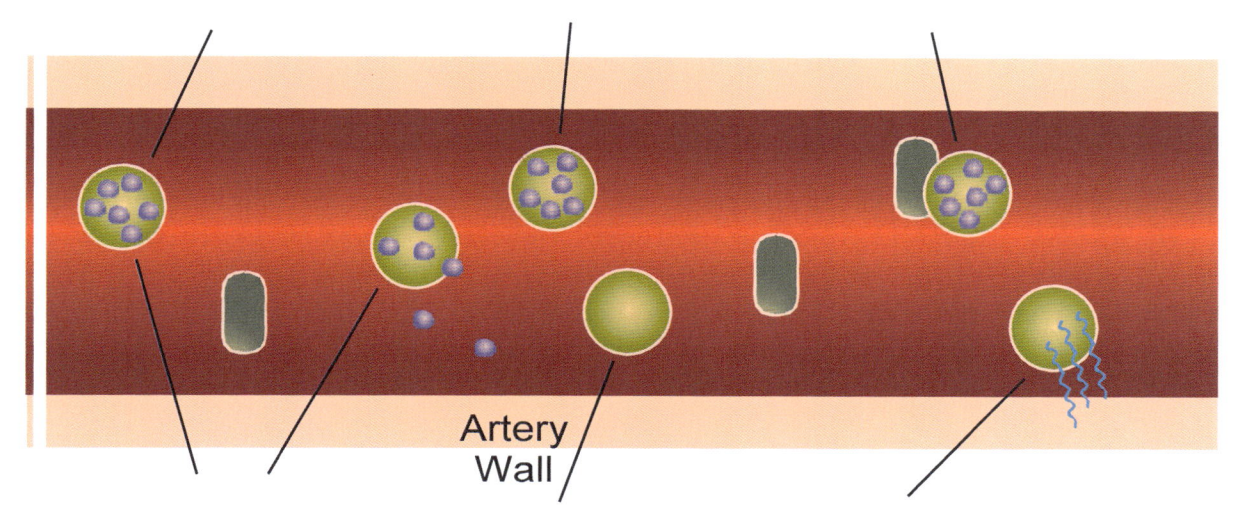

Artery Wall

VLDL's contain triglycerides which get dropped off and are used by the body for energy or stored as fat.

"Empty" VLDL's become LDL's.

Some LDL's are grabbed by protein receptors and pulled into the cells to perform work.

When things get out of balance...

The more saturated fat and cholesterol you eat, the more VLDL's are made in the liver.

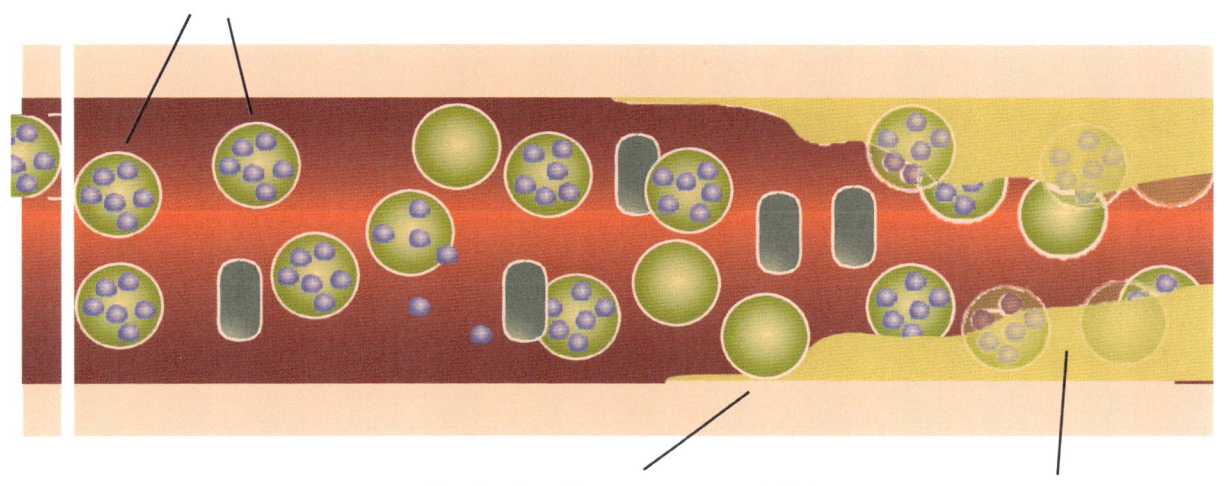

The body will not use more LDL's than necessary. Excess LDL's stick to blood vessel walls. Significant accumulation causes plaque.

Plaque build-up narrows the blood vessels and can lead to claudication.

Many clinical trials have shown the benefits of improving cholesterol in patients with PAD who also have heart disease or cerebral vascular disease, which causes strokes. The Heart Protection Study found that the lipid lowering drug simvastatin (a statin; see Chapter 8) reduced the risk of cardiovascular events over 5 years by 25% in a population of over 20,000 patients with atherosclerosis, of which 6,700 had PAD [1]. In addition, this study also showed a lower rate of angioplasty/stent or surgical bypass on lower extremities. Another study demonstrated that a statin decreased the incidence or worsening of intermittent claudication by 38% over 5.4 years [2]. Based on these findings, there are multiple benefits linked to reducing LDL cholesterol in PAD patients. These include decreased cardiovascular death, decreased rates of lower extremity complications needing angioplasty or surgery and a potential reduction in plaque formation in arteries. Some ways to reduce your bad cholesterol levels (LDL) are prescription medication from your physician, smoking cessation, diet and weight loss if you are over your ideal weight. Unfortunately, exercise does not significantly improve your LDL values, but will increase your good cholesterol (HDL) and decrease your triglyceride values. A more detailed description of medicines for high cholesterol is in chapter 8 of this book.

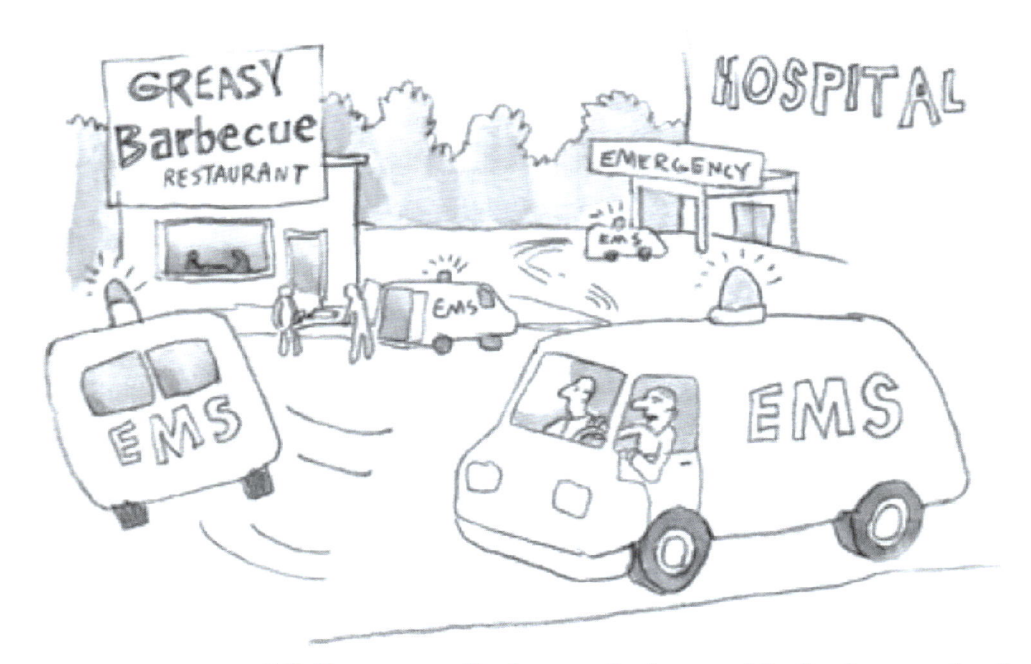

"Call me crazy. I'm just not in the mood for barbecue today."

New Guidelines and Recommendations

In 2014 the American Heart Association and the American College of Cardiology, along with the National Heart, Lung, and Blood Institute introduced new guidelines and recommendations for cholesterol [3]. The new guidelines no longer use LDL and HDL cholesterol targets. According to the expert panel, the reason for this is that there is no evidence from randomized, controlled clinical trials to support treatment to a specific value (e.g. LDL of < 100mg/dL). As a result, the new guidelines make no recommendations for specific LDL, HDL or triglyceride targets for prevention of atherosclerotic cardiovascular disease (ASCVD). Instead, the new guidelines identify 4 groups of patients to focus attention to reduce ASCVD events. The biggest change is that in these 4 patient groups, **the new guidelines focus on the use of statin drugs in order to achieve relative reductions in LDL cholesterol.**

The 4 groups of interest of can benefit from statin drugs are as follows:

- Individuals with known atherosclerotic cardiovascular disease (ASCVD)
- LDL-cholesterol levels >190 mg/dL
- Individuals with Diabetes
- Individuals without evidence of cardiovascular disease or diabetes but who have LDL-cholesterol levels between 70 and 189 mg/dL and a 10-year risk of atherosclerotic cardiovascular disease >7.5%

The dose of statin drugs for each group is dependent on age (older or younger than 75 years old) and risk profile (7.5% risk in 10 years), and is as follows:

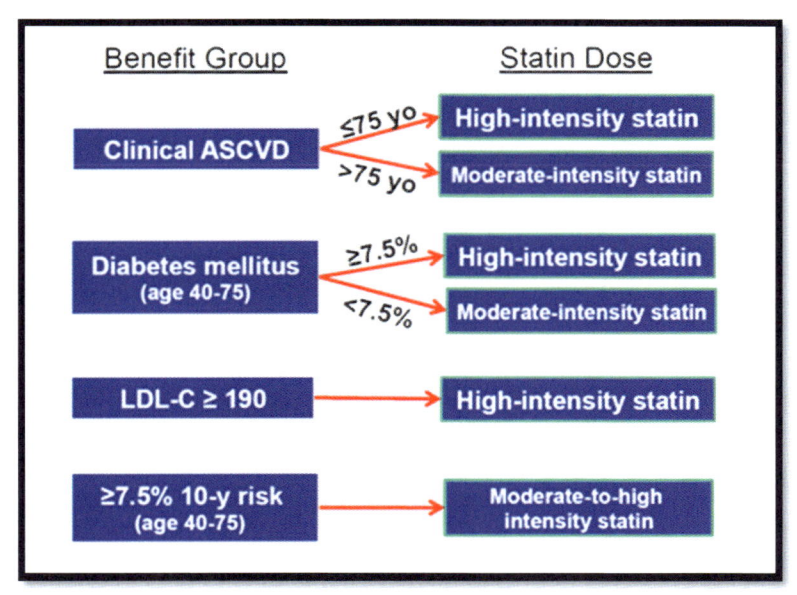

Benefit Group		Statin Dose
Clinical ASCVD	≤75 yo	High-intensity statin
	>75 yo	Moderate-intensity statin
Diabetes mellitus (age 40-75)	≥7.5%	High-intensity statin
	<7.5%	Moderate-intensity statin
LDL-C ≥ 190		High-intensity statin
≥7.5% 10-y risk (age 40-75)		Moderate-to-high intensity statin

The definition of statin dose is outlined in the table below:

High-Intensity Statin Therapy	Moderate-Intensity Statin Therapy	Low-Intensity Statin Therapy
Daily dose lowers LDL cholesterol by approximately ≥ 50%	Daily dose lowers LDL cholesterol by approximately 30% to < 50%	Daily dose lowers LDL cholesterol by approximately < 30%
Atorvastatin 40-80 mg Rosuvastatin 20-40 mg	Atorvastatin 10-20 mg Rosuvastatin 5-10 mg Simvastatin 20–40 mg Pravastatin 40-80 mg Lovastatin 40 mg Fluvastatin XL 80 mg Fluvastatin 40 mg BID Pitavastatin 2–4 mg	Simvastatin 10 mg Pravastatin 10–20 mg Lovastatin 20 mg Fluvastatin 20–40 mg Pitavastatin 1 mg

Recommendations Relative to PAD

- Have your cholesterol (lipid panel) checked routinely by your doctor.

- PAD is a form of atherosclerosis, and many PAD patients have diabetes. Therefore, all PAD patients should ask their doctor about being on a high to moderate dose of statin drugs.

- The American Heart Association, American College of Cardiology and the Inter-Society Consensus for the Management of Peripheral Arterial Disease recommend a LDL goal of < 100 mg/dL in patients with PAD; preferentially by using statin drugs. In higher risk PAD patients, a goal of < 70 mg/dL is recommended.

- Interestingly, evidence suggests that no atherosclerosis progression in the coronary arteries of the heart occurs after a concentration of 67 mg/dL is reached [4]. Currently, it is unknown if this is true for the lower extremity.

- Although not specifically addressed, it is important to also be aware of HDL and triglyceride levels. The higher your HDL levels the better. A value of 60 mg/dl is considered protective against atherosclerosis. If your triglycerides are 150 mg/dL or higher or HDL is less than 40 mg/dL, you should consult your doctor about a weight management and exercise training program. If you are smoking, STOP!

- If your triglycerides are 200–499 mg/dL, consult your physician on considering fibrate or niacin after lipid-lowering therapy.

- If your triglycerides are 500 mg/dL or higher, consult your physician on considering fibrate or niacin before LDL-lowering therapy. Consider omega-3 fatty acids as adjunct for high triglycerides.

Niacin (nicotinic acid) comes in prescription form and as "dietary supplements." Dietary supplement niacin is not regulated by the U.S. Food and Drug Administration (FDA) the same way that prescription niacin is. It may contain widely variable amounts of niacin — from none to much more than the label states. The amount of niacin may even vary from lot to lot of the same brand. Dietary supplement niacin must not be used as a substitute for prescription niacin. It should not be used for cholesterol lowering without consulting your doctor because of potentially very serious side effects. The use of resin is relatively contraindicated when triglycerides are over 200 mg/dL.

> **The most important thing to remember from this chapter:** Because having high levels of LDL and triglycerides or low values of HDL cholesterol are known to cause atherosclerosis, it is paramount that you have these checked regularly (yearly) by your doctor. If your values are undesirable, your doctor can prescribe medications and you can do other things such as exercise, lose weight, eat better, or stop smoking to reduce your risk of worsening PAD.

References

1) MRC/BHF Heart Protection Study of cholesterol lowering with simvastatin in 20,536 high risk individuals: A randomized placebo-controlled trial. 2002; Lancet. 360:7.
2) Pedersen TR, Kjekshus J, Pyorala K. Effect of simvstatin on ischemic signs and symptoms in the Scandinavian simvastatin survival study (4S). Am. J. Card. 1998; 81:333.

3) Stone NJ, Robinson JG, Lichtenstein AH, Bairey Merz CN, Blum CB, Eckel RH, Goldberg AC, Gordon D, Levy D, Lloyd-Jones DM, McBride P, Schwartz JS, Shero ST, Smith SC Jr, Watson K, Wilson PW; American College of Cardiology/American Heart Association Task Force on Practice Guidelines. 2013 ACC/AHA guideline on the treatment of blood cholesterol to reduce atherosclerotic cardiovascular risk in adults: a report of the American College of Cardiology/American Heart Association Task Force on Practice Guidelines. J Am Coll Cardiol. 2014;63(25 Pt B):2889-934.

4) O'Keefe JH Jr, Cordain L, Harris WH, Moe RM, Vogel R. Optimal low-density lipoprotein is 50 to 70 mg/dl: lower is better and physiologically normal. J Am Coll Cardiol. 2004;43(11):2142-6.

Chapter 6

Treatment Strategies: Adding Exercise to Your Life

Exercise has been shown to be one of the best therapies for PAD. **For long-term treatment, it may be better than any medicine or surgery.** Therefore, we have dedicated an entire chapter to exercise as a treatment. Patients with PAD often choose not to exercise because it hurts. Because walking for more than 3-4 minutes can be an excruciatingly painful endeavor, patients with PAD often cannot do what most take for granted such as shopping or yard work. Walking up hills can be especially painful. Unfortunately, over time they become more and more sedentary as the disease progresses and pain worsens. They eventually become trapped in their own homes and dependent on friends and relatives. This is not only a physical burden, but the loss of independence also weighs heavy on a patient's mind. By exercising regularly, you can prevent this gradual decline and maintain a quality of life.

Starting an Exercise Program

Congratulations if you have started an exercise program! Remember, although you will have good days and bad days, it is important to maintain your commitment to your exercise program in order to realize the benefits. Implementing a new activity into your life can be challenging. Don't worry, it is normal to have difficulties starting a new routine.

If you are contemplating starting exercise, first consult your doctor! It is recommended that a treadmill test be performed by your doctor before starting an exercise program. The treadmill test will screen you for any potential heart or blood pressure problems in addition to evaluating your leg pain and fitness level. As stated earlier, there is a strong relationship with PAD and heart problems. The information provided by this test will allow your doctor to evaluate you for any heart conditions that may be unknown. An exercise physiologist can prescribe a personal training program for you based on your claudication pain. **Ask your doctor if there is a local cardiac rehabilitation program or hospital based medically supervised exercise wellness center for you to join.** These programs provide additional support and health education. They also make it much more likely that you will stay with your exercise program and also make other good lifestyle changes. You will also meet others, like yourself, with similar conditions and find support and education in hearing their stories. Also, find out if your insurance covers this kind of program.

An important aspect of exercise adherence is developing and sticking to a routine. We recommend you get in the habit of exercising the same time of day, every day. It is recommended that you complete an exercise log each time you exercise. In this log you should write down how long you exercised, at what speed/elevation, how long it took for your legs to start hurting, and the total time or distance you walked, and any symptoms or comments you have. Use the form in this chapter to help you get started.

Unfortunately, many people who begin an exercise program are not exercising by the end of their first year. The good news is that with some planning, you can beat the drop-out odds and make a successful transition to a lifestyle that includes exercising regularly. Below are some suggestions that may help you:

Find a Supervised Program or a an Exercise Partner: Studies suggest that exercise adherence and improved walking benefits are greater if you are participating in a supervised program [1,2] or a family member or a friend is included in the commitment to exercise.

Make Sure You Complete Your Exercise Log or Journal: An exercise log or journal is an excellent way to look back and see how much progress you have made.

Schedule Your Workouts: Exercise must be a priority in order to establish it as a lifestyle practice. Make time for your workouts!

Wear Proper Clothing: Wear comfortable clothes appropriate for the environment (e.g. inside vs outside, hot weather vs cold weather). If walking, be sure to have comfortable shoes.

Take Your Mind Off It: One of the most used excuses for not exercising is boredom. Consider listening to your favorite music or books on tape to keep you entertained during your workout. Many pieces of exercise equipment have racks that fit onto the console to hold reading material. If you exercise at home, turn on some music or bring the television within viewing range. Rent a movie or tape and watch your favorite TV show while exercising. Or, call someone on your cell phone to pass the time while exercising. Call someone else who is exercising!

What Type of Exercise Should You Do? Although any kind of exercise is beneficial, there does appear to be an optimal training regimen for patients with PAD. It is best to walk at or near a pace that brings on leg pain within 10 minutes. Once pain begins, although difficult, it is best to walk as long as you are able to tolerate the pain before sitting down. Once the pain goes away with rest, you should get up and do this cycle again and again until you have completed 30 minutes of actual exercise time (walking time, not including rest time). These sessions should be performed approximately

> An alternative to structured exercise sessions is to purchase a physical activity tracker or pedometer and try to walk 5,000-10,000 steps a day. If you start at 5,000 steps per day and work your way up to 10,000 steps per day you will ensure that you achieve enough exercise to improve and maintain your walking ability. There are many devices on the market that can be bought, such as Fitbit, Apple Watch, Jawbone and Garmin. These devices can be interfaced with your smartphone or computer to chart your progress.

3 times a week. Remember, the pain you feel in your legs is a necessary occurrence to get maximal benefit from the walking. **Also remember this pain is not to be thought of as chest pain. If you get chest pain STOP EXERCISING IMMEDIATELY and call your doctor!** It is best to keep a training log to document what you did each day and bring it with you to your doctor visits. The following pages contain exercise worksheets that can get you started and give an example on how to document your exercise.

PAD Exercise Program Instructions

It is recommended that you walk at home or in a gym at least 3 days a week. Each exercise session should consist of 5 minutes of warm-up activities, 30 minutes of total walking time, and 5 minutes of cool-down activities. Begin your exercise session by performing 5 minutes of warm-up activities. You should begin walking and continue to do so until you reach a 4-5 on the leg pain scale. Once you have reached moderate to severe pain, stop and rest until your pain subsides. When you are ready to begin, walk again until you reach a 4-5 on the pain scale. Repeat this procedure until your total walking time reaches 30 minutes. Again, do not count your rest periods in this tally. Continue to walk and rest until you have walked a total of 30 minutes. Then, perform the cool-down movements.

If you are walking on a treadmill, you may find that walking at a specific grade and speed may get easier over time. If this is the case, increase your speed or the grade of the treadmill to challenge yourself as you progress.

1	No Pain
2	Onset of Pain
3	Mild Pain
4	Moderate Pain
5	Severe Pain

Log your activity (example logs are included in this chapter). Keep your logs as accurately as possible and show them to your doctor at your next appointment.

If you do not have access to a treadmill, you might want to walk in the mall so you can quickly find a bench or chair when the claudication pain becomes severe and you have to rest. Although any exercise is good, it is best to use walking as your exercise and not a stationary bike or other piece of equipment. This is because walking works the muscles in your calf, which are the most likely to be affected by PAD.

Do not give up if you do not see immediate results. Everyone has "good days" and "bad days" and improves at a different rate. Be consistent and patient. It usually takes 4-5 weeks before you will notice significant results. Remember, you must keep exercising, even after you start to feel better. The gained benefits will not be maintained if you stop. If you stop exercising, your legs will likely start to hurt again and you will quickly revert back to how you were feeling before you started the exercise program. You must make exercising 3 times week part of your lifestyle and make it a priority in your life!

What to Expect During a Single Exercise Session and the Training Effect of Repeated Exercise

At the beginning of each exercise session you can expect your heart rate to increase quickly, and then level off to a constant state. This initial increase is the body's way of meeting the demand of increased work required to exercise. By increasing your heart rate you gradually allow an increase of blood flow to working muscles, regulate your body's temperature (both warming the active muscles and joints and cooling the skin) and deliver oxygen and energy to muscles. This improves the muscle's flexibility, and prepares ligaments and tendons for exercise, thereby preventing muscle "pulls," strains, sprains and tightness, etc. You should always allow a warm-up period of 5 minutes prior to your prescribed exercise session. Proper warm-up will help prevent musculoskeletal injuries. A warm-up can be as simple as walking at a pace that is significantly slower than the pace you intend to use during your actual 30 minutes of exercise. For example, if 2.5 mph brings on leg pain in 5-6 minutes, then warm-up at 1.5 mph for 5 minutes before increasing the speed to 2.5 mph. Following this initial stage of warm-up, your body will settle into a rhythm with steady heart rate and breathing patterns. You should end each exercise session with a cool-down period similar to the warm-up period. This will prevent blood from pooling in your legs, prevent muscle soreness the next day, and decrease the risk of your heart not receiving enough oxygen immediately after exercise. It is important that you IMMEDIATELY document the exercise in your training log after exercise. It is a good idea to keep your training diary in the same spot and never move it. Make a conscious note to yourself when your next exercise training session will be and dedicate yourself to doing it.

How/When to Increase Walking

As your body becomes more conditioned, and your leg pain starts to decrease, you will be able to walk for longer time periods. It is not uncommon for a PAD patient to not be able to walk for more than 2 minutes initially. Remember, you want to walk at a speed or elevation that brings on pain. Therefore, as your legs get in better shape, the same speed, elevation and distance may not cause pain any more. You will need to periodically increase your workload (e.g. speed, elevation, distance) to initiate the leg pain. For example, you initially may start training at a walking speed of 2.0 mph and get leg pain after 3 minutes that is relieved after 2 minutes of rest. After 2 months of training, your leg pain may not occur or may occur only after 20 minutes. At that point, adjust the walking speed to 2.2 mph or slightly increase the elevation. Do not increase your workload too much too soon. Gradually "experiment" with small increases and allow time for your new claudication rate to "stabilize" before making a final decision. Your goal is to walk for 30-40 minutes 3 times a week at a speed that makes your legs hurt, but allows you to keep walking through the pain. If there is an interruption in training for more than 2-3 weeks for reasons such as vacation or illness, you may need to reduce your workload and work back up to where you were before the interruption.

EXERCISE LOG EXAMPLE

Day of Week	Exercise	Duration	Notes
Sunday	Walked at mall	12 minutes briskly Rest 3 minutes 10 minutes briskly Rest 2 minutes 8 minutes slow Total 30 minutes	Right calf pain 5/5 each time I stopped Total steps for day: 5,312
	Exercise	Duration	Notes
Monday	Walked on treadmill	15 minutes at 2.5 mph Rest 5 minutes 17 minutes at 2.2 mph Total 32 minutes	Walked faster than when at the mall Total steps for day: 6,789
	Exercise	Duration	Notes
Tuesday	Walked outside after dinner	25 minutes slowly	Going up hills hurt leg 4/5 Total steps for day: 6,100
	Exercise	Duration	Notes
Wednesday	Walked outside in the morning	35 minutes at brisk pace	Legs felt good today Total steps for day: 8,200
	Exercise	Duration	Notes
Thursday	Walked on treadmill	15 minutes at 2.5 mph Rest 5 minutes 17 minutes at 2.2 mph Total 32 minutes	Walked faster than when at the mall Total steps for day: 7,500
	Exercise	Duration	Notes
Friday	Did not exercise, but went shopping and walked a lot		Total steps for day: 8,842
	Exercise	Duration	Notes
Saturday	Rest day		Total steps for day: 2,107

BLANK EXERCISE LOG

Day of Week	Exercise	Duration	Notes
Sunday			
Monday			
Tuesday			
Wednesday			
Thursday			
Friday			
Saturday			

Recognition of Symptoms

Although exercise and physical exertion may cause some general discomfort, it is important to recognize the difference between normal pain and dangerous symptoms related to heart disease. If you learn the warning signs of heart problems and what steps to take, you can prevent most dangerous situations. Below is a list of normal and potentially abnormal symptoms to consider when exercising:

Normal Responses

Leg Pain (claudication): It is normal for patients with PAD to get claudication after 3-4 minutes of exercise. Try to push through this pain until it is moderate to severe. Rest until the pain goes away, and then begin exercising again.

Increased Breathing: It is normal for your breathing to increase in rate and depth while exercising. This increase will be more noticeable at the start of exercise and then become more comfortable after 3-5 minutes of exercise.

Sweating: While exercising your body will begin to perspire for the purpose of regulating your body's temperature (cooling you down).

Leg Muscle Burning: You may experience some burning/fatigue sensation in your legs. This is a normal response of a muscle that is not used to exercising. You may also experience some delayed muscle soreness 2-3 days following exercise. This will begin to lessen as your fitness increases.

Joint Pain/Stiffness: Although pain in your knees, ankles, hips, etc. will likely occur, it is important that you do not "overdo it" and cause an injury that keeps you from exercising. Allowing a 5 minute warm-up period will help reduce this risk. Stop exercising if you experience any sharp shooting pains or have pain that causes you to walk abnormally (e.g. limp). Please contact your physician if any abnormal swelling occurs following exercise. Over the counter Tylenol usually alleviates this type of pain. Consult your physician before taking any new medication.

Abnormal Responses

Chest Discomfort: Most heart attacks involve discomfort in the center of the chest that lasts for more than a few minutes, or goes away and comes back. The discomfort can feel like uncomfortable pressure, squeezing, fullness, or pain.

Discomfort in Other Areas of the Upper Body: Pain or discomfort from the heart will often radiate into in one or both arms, the back, neck, or jaw.

Shortness of Breath: The feeling of not getting enough air or having difficulty catching your breath at rest or after stopping exercise often occurs with chest discomfort. But it also can occur before chest discomfort.

Other Warning Symptoms. May include breaking out in a cold sweat, nausea, severe headache, loss of coordination, light-headedness/dizziness or joint/bone/muscle pain that is not relieved with rest.

General Benefits of Exercise

The recommendation for regular exercise to prevent and treat PAD, heart disease, or diabetes and provide other health benefits is accepted throughout the medical community. Along with taking your medication and managing your lifestyle, patients with known PAD can benefit greatly from regular exercise. Below is a list of how regular exercise can improve your general health in addition to your PAD specific problems.

more than 50 studies have shown that exercise is beneficial for PAD patients

Cardiovascular Benefits

- **Improve the body's ability to take in, deliver and use oxygen to organs and muscles.** This is related to how long you can walk and is generally accepted as the best measurement of physical fitness.

- **Lower heart rate** at rest and at low levels of exertion and exercise. This is accomplished by increasing the amount of blood which is pumped per heartbeat. The hearts of fit people do not work as hard as unfit people at rest or during light to moderate activities.

- **Lower blood pressure.** The amount of force exerted on your vessels is decreased both during contraction (systolic) and between beats (diastolic) following exercise training. High blood pressure is a risk for PAD, coronary artery disease, stroke, and diabetes.

- **Blood lipids.** Regular exercise increases "good cholesterol" (HDL), and reduces triglycerides.

- **Body composition.** Exercise helps prevent weight gain, reduces the percent of fat on your body, and increases muscle. With proper nutrition planning, exercise can aid in weight loss.

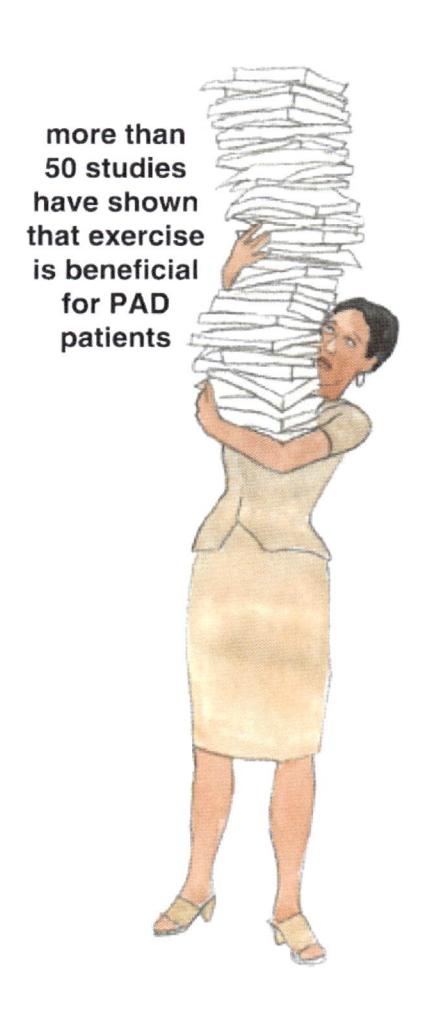

Musculoskeletal Benefits

- Regular exercise makes the muscles of PAD patients more efficient at using the blood and oxygen they receive
- It is believed that exercise can elicit the growth of new blood vessels in the muscle of PAD patients
- Increase muscle strength and endurance (many PAD patients have a loss of muscle mass due to physical inactivity)
- Improve flexibility
- Prevent injury by improving reaction time
- Helps prevent losses in bone density, thereby preventing osteoporosis and fractures during accidents or falls
- Increase coordination and balance
- Improve insulin sensitivity and glucose (sugar) tolerance to prevent or improve diabetes

Psychological Benefits

- Decrease stress/anxiety and improve your ability to manage or cope with stress/anxiety
- Reduce depression by creating positive self-esteem, image and confidence
- Improve ability to relax, reduce irritability and hostility
- Improve ability to fall asleep and make sleep more restful
- Improve alertness and concentration
- Gain a positive, happy, optimistic outlook on life

Other Benefits

- Help prevent certain cancers (e.g. colon, prostate, breast, uterine)
- Improve social opportunities
- Gain discipline of a goal oriented, structured, dedicated, organized program.

Safety

Eating Before Exercise. Eat approximately 60-90 minutes before exercising. This will give your body time to digest food and provide enough energy for the exercise. Exercising in the very early morning after an overnight fast may cause dizziness. Exercising too soon after eating may cause stomach pain or cramps, or a bloated feeling. If you are diabetic, check your blood glucose before exercising for a safe level.

Always start with a warm-up and end with a cool-down. Your body needs time to adjust to an exercise challenge and time to cool-down after the challenge. These guidelines are outlined in a previous section. Never start exercising on an incline, at a fast speed or difficult pedal workload. The main point to remember is to allow 5 minutes before and after your exercise session to walk or bike at a very easy workload.

General Considerations. Try not to exercise alone. If you do go for a walk alone, tell someone when and where you are going. If you have heart disease, do not exercise above your specified heart rate zone prescribed to you by your doctor. Maintain a training log. Increase your speed and time gradually. It is important that you contact your doctor if your health changes. For example, let your doctor know if you visit the emergency room, have an extended illness causing you to stop exercise for more than 2-3 weeks, are hospitalized, or hurt yourself exercising.

Environmental Conditions

It is preferred that you exercise on a treadmill at home or inside a mall or wellness center with benches rather than a bicycle. However, if on occasion you walk outside be careful to avoid extreme hot humid or cold temperatures. Do not exercise on days with high pollutant indexes provided by the TV news. **For most PAD patients walking up hills or walking outside will cause more leg pain than flat surfaces or indoor treadmills at zero elevation.** For this reason, be aware of where you will be walking and have a plan to sit down if necessary. For example, malls and parks usually have benches to sit on. Do not take an extremely hot or cold shower immediately following exercise. These temperature extremes may dilate or constrict your vessels and could cause fainting. Last, be sure to stay hydrated by drinking plenty of water.

Why Does Exercise Work?

Clinicians have long appreciated that exercise in general can prevent or help treat numerous diseases. In PAD, it is likely that exercise decreases leg pain by stimulating formation of new small blood vessels, called capillaries, in skeletal muscle, a process known as angiogenesis [3,4]. It has been suggested that because an artery is blocked, the body will actually grow a new blood vessel to go around (or bypass) the blocked area. This is called collateral development. If you have been sedentary, exercise training will also improve your heart's pumping capacity, increase arterial vasodilation (making it more efficient for blood to travel) and increase the amount of blood that returns to your heart. All of these beneficial adaptations due to exercise training will improve your functional capacity.

> **The most important thing to remember from this chapter:** Regular exercise offers many health benefits. It can help you enjoy a better quality of life by allowing you to do things for a longer period of time without having to stop due to leg pain. It is best to walk at or near a pace that brings on leg pain within 10 minutes. Once pain begins, it is best to walk as long as you are able to tolerate the pain. Once the pain goes away with rest, you should do this cycle again and again until you have completed 30 minutes of actual exercise time. These sessions should be performed at least 3 times a week.

References

1) Fokkenrood HJ, Bendermacher BL, Lauret GJ, Willigendael EM, Prins MH, Teijink JA. Supervised exercise therapy versus non-supervised exercise therapy for intermittent claudication. Cochrane Database Syst Rev. 2013 23;8:CD005263.
2) Vemulapalli S, Dolor RJ, Hasselblad V, Schmit K, Banks A, Heidenfelder B, Patel MR, Jones WS. Supervised vs unsupervised exercise for intermittent claudication: A systematic review and meta-analysis. Am Heart J. 2015; 169(6):924-937.
3) Duscha BD1, Robbins JL, Jones WS, Kraus WE, Lye RJ, Sanders JM, Allen JD, Regensteiner JG, Hiatt WR, Annex BH. Angiogenesis in skeletal muscle precede improvements in peak oxygen uptake in peripheral artery disease patients. Arterioscler Thromb Vasc Biol. 2011; 31(11):2742-8.
4) Haas TL1, Lloyd PG, Yang HT, Terjung RL. Exercise training and peripheral arterial disease. Compr Physiol. 2012; 2(4):2933-3017.

Chapter 7
Treatment Strategies: Lifestyle Management of Hypertension, Weight and Diet

Hypertension (High Blood Pressure)

Having high blood pressure makes your heart work harder than normal and causes damage to the inside of your arteries. **The medical term for high blood pressure is hypertension.** The two words high blood pressure and hypertension mean the same thing. **It is desirable to have a blood pressure of 120/80 or lower.** You are considered to have hypertension if your blood pressure reading is greater than 140/90. The top number is your "systolic" pressure and is related to pressure when your heart beats while the bottom number is your "diastolic" pressure which is related to the pressure when your heart is relaxed between beats. Unfortunately, elevated blood pressure has no symptoms; therefore you may have it but never know it. Because of this, it is a good idea to have your blood pressure checked routinely, at least 2-3 times a year. Try to have it taken at the same time of day after resting for a while. If any reading appears to be higher than usual, you should monitor it closely for a couple of weeks to see if it is consistently high. One isolated high measurement does not indicate you have hypertension, however consistently high values over a period of time may require medical attention. The table on the next page shows the significance of a variety of blood pressure readings. Which one do you fall into?

Classifying Your Blood Pressure

The reason why hypertension contributes to atherosclerosis, stroke and PAD is that it injures the walls of arteries causing plaque build-up and making the artery hard and stiff. Although this affects all arteries, it is of particular importance to the renal arteries. High blood pressure is one of the primary causes of kidney failure. Although it has not been proven that maintaining normal blood pressure decreases cardiovascular events, it is unknown if antihypertensive therapy prevents the worsening of PAD.

Blood Pressure Classifications

Systolic	Diastolic	Classification
Less than 130	Less than 85	Normal
130 to 139	85 to 89	High Normal
140 to 159	90 to 99	Stage 1 Mild Hypertension
160 to 179	100 to 109	Stage 2 Moderate Hypertension
180 or Greater	110 or Greater	Stage 3 Severe Hypertension

Blood Pressure Control

Goal:

- Systolic BP less than 140/90 mm Hg
- Systolic BP less than 130/80 mm Hg in people with diabetes, heart failure or renal (kidney) insufficiency

Intervention Recommendations

- Become more physically active. A regular exercise routine is beneficial for lowering blood pressure.
- Try to lose weight or maintain your optimal weight.
- Reduce the amount of sodium (salt) in your diet and eat a low fat diet rich in fruit, vegetables and whole grains.
- Only drink alcohol in moderation.
- Try to limit the amount of stress in your life. Make time for yourself and relax.
- Don't smoke! Smoking causes your blood vessels to get smaller (constrict) and your heart to beat faster-two things that raise your blood pressure
- Consult your doctor about what medications (e.g. beta-blockers and ACE inhibitors) are available if lifestyle changes do not reduce your blood pressure

High Blood Pressure Statistics [1]

- High blood pressure (hypertension) kills approximately 50,000 Americans each year. According to the American Heart Association, it was listed as a primary or contributing cause of death in > 250,000 U.S. deaths
- As many as 65 million Americans age 6 and older have high blood pressure
- Nearly 1 in 3 adults in the U.S. has high blood pressure
- More than 40% of African Americans have high blood pressure
- 30% of people with high blood pressure don't know they have it because there are no symptoms and people do not have their blood pressure checked regularly
- The cause of 90–95% of the cases of high blood pressure isn't known, however high blood pressure is easily detected and usually controllable

Weight Management

Body weight may be directly related to the distance a PAD patient can walk before getting claudication pain. Therefore, overweight individuals who lose weight can enjoy improved walking distances and a better quality of life. Obesity is also recognized as a risk factor for many other diseases, including cardiovascular disease, which is the number one enemy of PAD patients. The most effective way to lose weight is through diet and exercise. First, determine what your ideal weight should be based on your height. This is done by using a BMI (Body Mass Index) table (next page). Your goal should be a BMI of 18.5–24.9 kg/m^2. (BMI of 25 corresponds to 110 percent of desirable body weight. People with a BMI of 25–29.9 are considered overweight, while people with a BMI of 30 or greater are considered obese.) Second, measure your waist circumference. Men should have a measurement of less than 40 inches and women less than 35 inches. This simple measurement has been proven to show who is at a higher risk of disease progression.

Diet

Although weight loss itself is very difficult, the concept is very easy. If you burn more calories than you take in, you will lose weight. Therefore, decreasing the amount of calories you eat and increasing the physical activity should allow you to gradually take off unwanted pounds. We recommend taking an honest look at what types of foods you eat.

BODY MASS INDEX CHART

Weight (pounds)

Body Mass Index	58	59	60	61	62	63	64	65	66	67	68	69	70	71	72	73	74
19	91	94	97	100	104	107	110	114	118	121	125	128	132	136	140	144	148
20	96	99	102	106	109	113	116	120	124	127	131	135	139	143	147	151	155
21	100	104	107	111	115	118	122	126	130	134	138	142	146	150	154	159	163
22	105	109	112	116	120	124	128	132	136	140	144	149	153	157	162	166	171
23	110	114	118	122	126	130	134	138	142	146	151	155	160	165	169	174	179
24	115	119	123	127	131	135	140	144	148	153	158	162	167	172	177	182	186
25	119	124	128	132	136	141	145	150	155	159	164	169	174	179	184	189	194
26	124	128	133	137	142	146	151	156	161	166	171	176	181	186	191	197	202
27	129	133	138	143	147	152	157	162	167	172	177	182	188	193	199	204	210
28	134	138	143	148	153	158	163	168	173	178	184	189	195	200	206	212	218
29	138	143	148	153	158	163	169	174	179	185	190	196	202	208	213	219	225
30	143	148	153	158	164	169	174	180	186	191	197	203	209	215	221	227	233
31	148	153	158	164	169	175	180	186	192	198	203	209	216	222	228	235	241
32	153	158	163	169	175	180	186	192	198	204	210	216	222	229	235	242	249
33	158	163	168	174	180	186	192	198	204	211	216	223	229	236	242	250	256
34	162	168	174	180	186	191	197	204	210	217	223	230	236	243	250	257	264
35	167	173	179	185	191	197	204	210	216	223	230	236	243	250	258	265	272

Height (inches)

SOURCE: National Heart, Lung, and Blood Institute.

Good Choice	Bad Choice
Water Reduced calorie juices Diet soda (in moderation)	Coffee drinks Sweet fruit juices Sugary sodas Sport drinks Beer, dessert wine, hard liquor
Lean red meats Skinless, white-meat poultry Any fresh fish, especially cold-water fish high in "omega-3 fatty acids (salmon, tuna, black cod, herring). Dried beans + peas (lima, kidney, split peas, black-eyed peas, lentils) Soybeans and soy products, for example, soy burgers	Fatty marbled red meat Any fried, smoked, breaded or canned meats Processed meats (hotdogs, luncheon meats, bacon, sausage) Organ meats, such as liver Fast food sandwiches Refried beans Shellfish (shrimp, crab, lobster, clams, oyster)
Fat-free or low-fat dairy products, such as yogurt and cheese Skim or low-fat (1 percent) milk Egg whites or egg substitutes	Full-fat milk Egg yolks, butter, mayonaise Heavy cream sauces
In season fresh or frozen fruit and vegetables Low-sodium canned vegetables Canned fruit packed in juice or water	Fried or breaded vegetables High sodium canned vegetables Canned fruit packed in heavy syrup
Whole grains + cereals (100% whole wheat bread, brown rice, oatmeal, 100% whole grain/wheat crackers) Nuts (in moderation) Whole-wheat flour High-fiber cereal with 5 or more grams of fiber per serving Whole-grain pasta Oatmeal	Refined grains + cereals (white bread or rice, processed cereals, white pastas) Most breakfast cereals and granola bars Packaged noodles/rice with sauce Bakery items (cakes, pies, cookies, pies, doughnuts, muffins, pastries, brownies, quick breads) Corn bread, biscuits, egg noodles, high-fat snack crackers , chips
Canola oil or olive oil Margarine made with liquid oil rather than trans fat Cholesterol-lowering margarine	Butter, lard, bacon grease Gravies and heavy cream sauces Hydrogenated margarine and shortening Cocoa butter, found in chocolate Coconut, palm and palm kernel oils

Try to avoid high fat foods such as fast food restaurants or fried foods and empty calories such as sugary soda pop. Concentrate on fruits and vegetables, whole grains and lean meats. Last, although some special diets have shown to be beneficial, consult your doctor before starting any diet other than a low fat diet. Below is a list of 50 tips and considerations that can help you eat a low fat, heart healthy and PAD friendly diet.

Last, when planning a weight loss program, it is important to remember some "approximate" values. You have to burn about 3,500 calories to lose 1 pound. This equation is not perfect and can be subtly different from individual to individual due to metabolism, but does serve as a general rule. So, based on this general calculation, if you expend 500 more calories than you take in each day, you should lose about 1 pound a week (500 calories x 7 days = 3,500 calories). This is best accomplished by decreasing the calories you consume in your daily diet. However, you can also increase the amount of calories burned by exercising. Whether you walk or run a mile, the calories burned comes out relatively the same (walking very fast or running expends about 15-20% more calories than slow walking); about 100 ± 20 calories. So, if you decreased your diet by 400 calories per day and you walked 1 mile a day, this combination of diet and exercise would still achieve a daily caloric value of (-) 500 calories (400 from diet and 100 from exercise = 500 calories total). It is best to decrease your dietary calories by 400-750 calories per day and increase your daily physical activity by 100-250 calories per day to achieve a weight loss of 1-2 pounds per week. It is also recommended to consult a nutritionist for meal planning strategies.

50 additional helpful ideas to keep weight off:

1) Never go grocery shopping hungry
2) Do not eat if you are not hungry
3) Avoid eating after 8:00pm
4) Eat a light breakfast instead of skipping breakfast
5) Snack smart: fruit, popcorn (no butter), low-fat yogurt
6) Try to maintain a regular sleep schedule
7) Do not lose more than 2-3 pounds per week
8) Eat smaller portions and avoid family style meals and buffets
9) Remember that alcoholic beverages give you empty calories
10) Avoid cream sauces/soups and gravies
11) Do not eat chicken/turkey skin
12) Drink skim milk versus whole milk or low fat
13) Remember creamy salad dressings often are high in calories
14) Cook with canola oil, it has the lowest amount of saturated fat (7%)
15) Eat slowly to allow your brain to tell you when you are full

16) Avoid drinks high in sugar and low in nutrition like soda or fruit drinks
17) When eating out, do NOT think you have to eat everything on your plate
18) Take a walk after eating
19) Do NOT skip meals, especially breakfast!
20) Grocery shop from a list, DO NOT buy spontaneously
21) Plan meals
22) Use a food scale at home- one serving of meat is 4 oz!
23) Avoid vending machines
24) When cooking, substitute 1 C plain yogurt for 1 C sour cream in dressings and sauces- you'll reduce by 350 fewer calories, 44 fewer grams of total fat, and nearly 28 fewer grams of saturated fat!!
25) When cooking, try lemon juice/herbs instead of butter or heavy sauces
26) Trim all visible fat from your meat
27) Try not to eat any red meat one day a week
28) When baking, substitute 2 egg whites for every whole egg
29) If you must order an appetizer, avoid breaded and fried foods
30) Make an effort to eat fish twice a month
31) Choose white meat over dark meat—dark meat has twice the calories!
32) When selecting ground meat from the grocer-read the label and choose the lower fat brand
33) Avoid or minimally salt your food
34) Take the stairs vs the elevator
35) Buy a pedometer and log the steps you take per day. Try and increase the steps over time.
36) Do not leave snacks out in the open
37) Do not open the refrigerator unless you have a reason
38) When dining out, split an entrée or dessert with someone
39) When baking, substitute apple sauce for fatty oils
40) Eat more fiber and bulk foods like bran, fruits and vegetables to make you feel full
41) If at a party, "dip" raw vegetables vs chips, crackers, etc.
42) Pack a sensible lunch for work to avoid going out to eat
43) When thirsty, add a twist of lemon/lime to water instead of drinking a sugary soda or fruit drink
44) Walk your dog more often—this will be good for you AND your dog!
45) If you are exercising, exercise at the same time of day every day. Keep your routine.
46) Avoid exotic coffee drinks—a café white chocolate mocha contains 440 calories!!! You would have to walk/run over 4 miles to burn that off!!
47) Seek the support of those around you. Don't be afraid or embarrassed to ask them to keep you motivated.
48) Drink an extra glass of water per day

49) Avoid fad diets
50) Do not think of yourself as dieting; think of it as a new lifestyle.

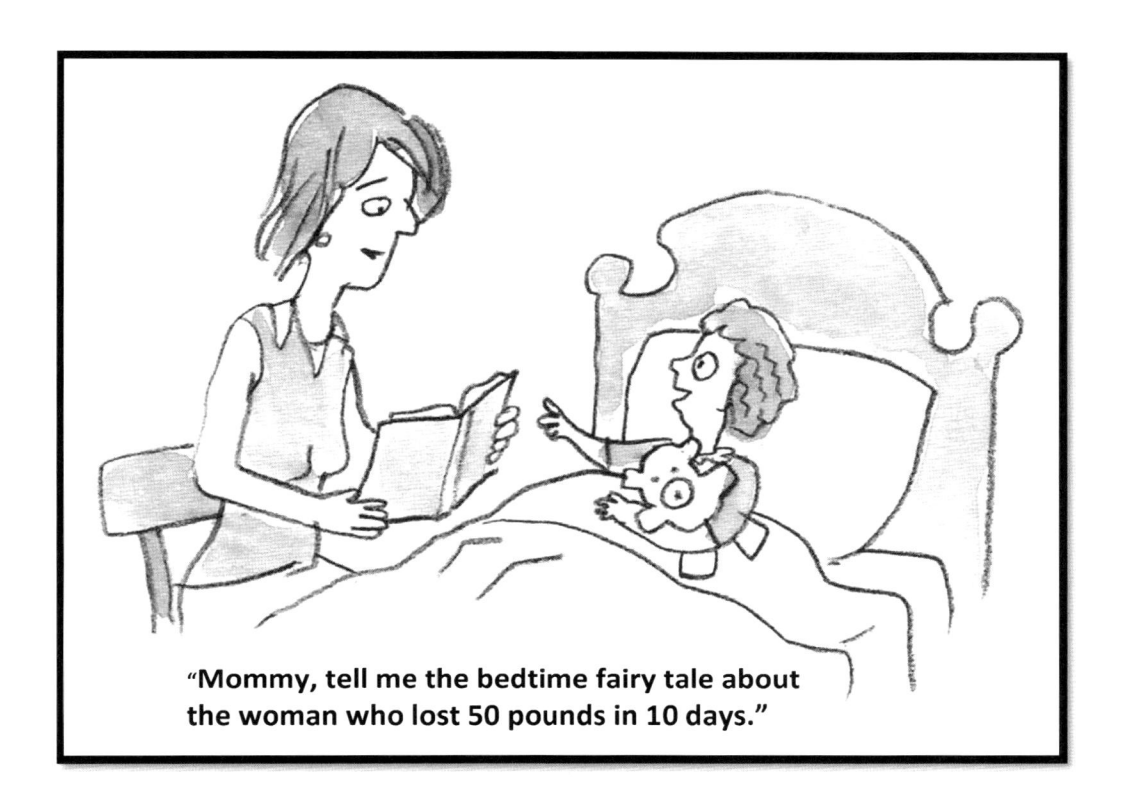

"Mommy, tell me the bedtime fairy tale about the woman who lost 50 pounds in 10 days."

The most important thing to remember from this chapter: Controlling your blood pressure, eating healthy and maintaining a healthy weight can help you manage your PAD. Try to lower your blood pressure to 120/80 and have it checked at least twice a year. You can lower your blood pressure by exercising, weight loss, eating a low salt diet, avoiding stress, medication or smoking cessation. Many people do not worry about high blood pressure, because it is painless, until it is too late. The most effective way to lose weight is to eat better foods and fewer calories. Take time to understand good and bad food choices and be diligent in practicing this every day. Set a reasonable goal of 1-2 pounds of weight loss per week for a month and then try adding an exercise program to expend additional calories.

References

1) Heart disease and stroke statistics--2015 update: a report from the American Heart Association.

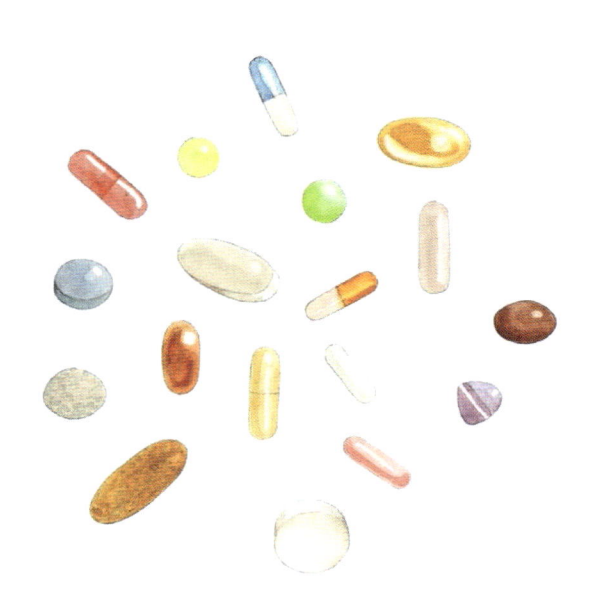

Chapter 8

Treatment Strategies: Medications to Consider

One of the first steps in treating PAD is to optimize your medication to control risk factors for atherosclerosis. Therefore, patients with PAD should be considered as candidates for medication that control blood pressure and diabetes, prevent blood from clotting, dilate (open) blood vessels, and reduce cholesterol. Two of the most important medications for treating PAD are called statins (and other lipid lowering medications) and anti-platelet drugs. A brief description of each is provided below. Each medication has a generic name and a trade/brand name. For example, simvastatin is the generic name for Zocor. In this chapter we will list the name given by the manufacturer followed by the generic name in parentheses e.g. Zocor (simvastatin). As with all medications, it is important to check with your doctor for contraindications due to other health conditions, interactions with other drugs you are taking or if you are, or are planning to become pregnant. No one should begin a new drug either over the counter or prescription without a consultation visit with their doctor.

Statins (HMG-CoA reductase inhibitors)

Examples: Lipitor (atorvastatin), Zocor (simvastatin), Lescol (fluvastatin), Mevacor (lovastatin), Pravachol (pravastatin), Crestor (rosuvastatin)

How They Work: Statins have a number of beneficial effects. First, statin drugs lower bad LDL cholesterol better than any other drug. Because of this, the statins have become one of the most widely prescribed drugs for patients with any type of atherosclerosis (heart disease, PAD or stroke). They work by preventing an enzyme, called HMG-CoA reductase, from working that regulates the production of cholesterol in the body. Less of this enzyme results in less cholesterol production. A second reason statin drugs are believed to work is that they stabilize the fragile plaque on the inside of arteries. By stabilizing the plaque it prevents a rupture and a blockage by a clot (thrombosis). Third, statins also decrease triglycerides and increase the good HDL cholesterol. It is best to take statins in the evening before you go to bed. This is when the body produces the most cholesterol. In addition, statins may have the potential to improve walking ability.

Clinical Trial Evidence: Several studies have shown statins to be beneficial for treating vascular diseases [1,2,3]. Statins usually reduce bad LDL cholesterol by 20-60% after 4-6 weeks of usage. Several clinical trials in patients with PAD have shown both a decrease in death and heart attack in patients who take statin drugs. For example, Zocor (simvastatin) has been shown to lower cardiovascular events in patients with PAD who had low LDL even prior to beginning statin therapy [4]! One study in patients with PAD has showed that 6 months of simvastatin therapy improved pain-free walking, total walking distance, and ABI's [5]. The Scandinavian Simvastatin Survival Study (4S) found that simvastatin decreased the risk of developing new or worsening claudication by 38% versus placebo [6]. Another large clinical trial showed that use of 80 mg/day of atorvastatin increased pain free walking by 60% and increased activity patterns of patients with claudication after one year [7].

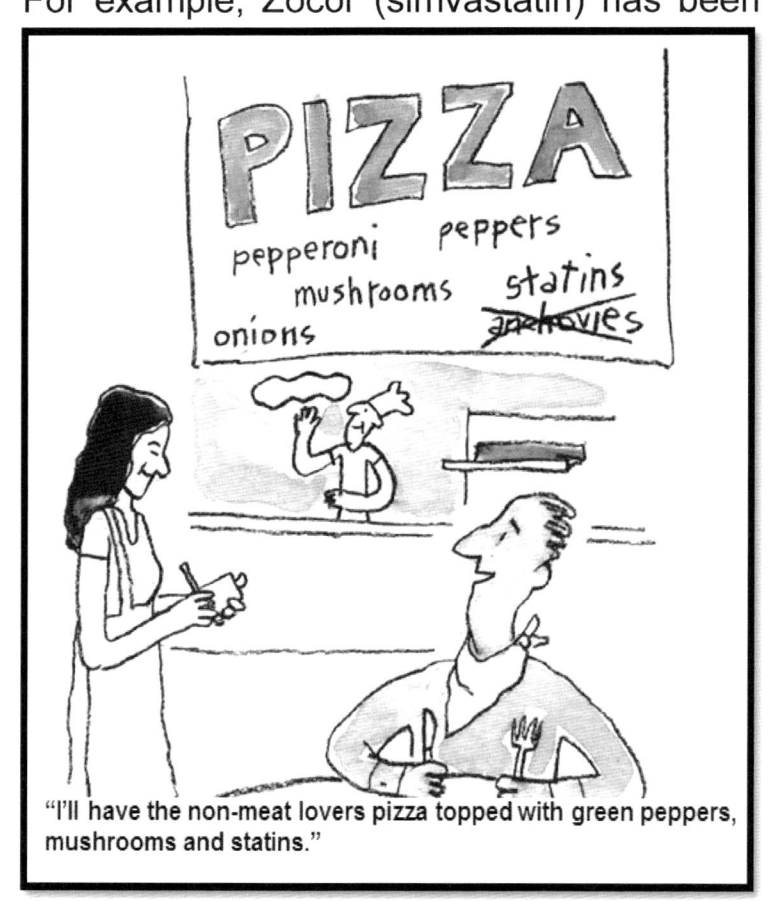

"I'll have the non-meat lovers pizza topped with green peppers, mushrooms and statins."

Safety, Potential Contraindications/Interactions: Statins are well tolerated by most patients. However, your doctor will draw your blood after 6-8 weeks of usage and periodically thereafter to make sure no unwanted side effects are occurring, such as liver damage. The most common side effects include an upset stomach, abdominal cramps, and constipation. Although uncomfortable, these generally go away as your body gets used to the medicine. Some patients experience muscle weakness, pain or soreness. You should contact your doctor if any of the above side effects occur.

Antiplatelet Agents/Anticoagulants/Blood Thinners

Examples: Aspirin, Plavix (clopidogral) and Coumadin (warfarin)

How They Work: Under normal conditions when someone injures themselves (e.g. accidentally cutting yourself) the blood forms a clot to stop the bleeding. While this process is essential to healing, the formation of blood clots can be dangerous in some situations. A "bad" blood clot occurs when cells in the blood called platelets clump together where plaque forms in a blood vessel. If a blood clot is formed inside a blood vessel, often as a response to injury to the vessel such as occurs with atherosclerosis, it raises the risk of heart attack or stroke. This may occur when a blood clot grows large enough to block a blood vessel (thrombus), or a piece of clot breaks off, travels through the bloodstream and blocks a blood vessel in another part of the body (embolism). To help prevent this, physicians may prescribe antiplatelets, which inhibit platelet's clotting activity. Antiplatelets are types of anticoagulants – medications used to help prevent the formation of blood clots when no injury has occurred. Antiplatelet agents work by preventing these platelets in the blood from clumping. In simple terms, they make your blood less "sticky."

Clinical Trial Evidence: In a study looking at 145 randomized trials with 9,214 patients with PAD, antiplatelet drugs were found to reduce the risk of heart attack, stroke or death by 22% [8]. The most common and most cost effective antiplatelet therapy is a daily 81 mg pill of baby aspirin. However, a study has shown taking Plavix instead of aspirin was 24% better for reducing cardiovascular and cerebrovascular events in 6,452 patients with PAD [9]. In combination with aspirin a recent study showed that taking aspirin combined with Plavix for unstable angina or heart attack reduced the risk of death, another heart attack, or stroke by 20% [10]. However, this finding is questioned by some who argue there is no evidence to support taking a combination of Plavix and aspirin versus a single antiplatelet drug alone for patients with lower extremity PAD. Due to potential side effects, it is necessary to discuss these medications with your physician and be monitored regularly. There is strong evidence that shows antiplatelet drugs also prevent blockages in arteries after revascularization surgery (vein bypass graft) by approximately 40% [8]. Given the many benefits of antiplatelet (aspirin) and anticoagulant (Coumadin) therapies separately, it seems logical that a combination of the two might be even better. However, researchers have found that a combination of low-dose Coumadin and low-dose aspirin is no more effective than aspirin by itself. Furthermore, in the study group, major bleeding episodes (primarily gastrointestinal) occurred nearly twice as often in the combination-therapy patients compared with the aspirin-only patients.

Safety, Potential Contraindications/Interactions: Plavix has been evaluated for safety in more than 11,300 patients, including over 7,000 patients treated for 1 year or more. The overall tolerability of Plavix was similar to that of aspirin regardless of age, gender and race, with an approximately equal incidence (13%) of patients withdrawing from treatment because of adverse reactions. The most likely adverse effects of antiplatelet therapy include: internal bleeding, abdominal pain/constipation, and skin rash and bruising. Potential or unknown drug interactions may occur when taken in combination with heparin, non-steroidal anti-inflammatory drugs (NSAIDs), or beta-blocking agents. Because of the risk for internal bleeding, you should immediately call your doctor if you experience bloody/black stools, blood in your urine or unusual abdominal pain. Last, be extremely cautious about taking any herbal remedies and diet supplements if you are on an anticoagulant. A wide assortment of herbal products, including St. John's Wort, coenzyme Q10, garlic, ginkgo biloba and vitamin K are known to interact with coumadin or otherwise affect coagulation.

Other Medications to Consider

Depending on the severity of your PAD and the known amount of atherosclerosis in other parts of your body, like coronary heart disease, your doctor may prescribe other medicines in addition to statins and antiplatelets. **Currently, two drugs have been FDA approved and recommended for some patients with claudication. These drugs are Trental (pentoxifylline) and Pletal (cilostazol).** Trental works by decreasing blood viscosity and changing the shape of blood cells as they pass through narrow spaces such as blood vessels. By doing so, this drug allows blood to flow more freely and deliver more oxygen to your muscles. It has also been shown to improve pain free walking [11,12]. Pletal works by vasodilating blood vessels and preventing blood from clotting. Pletal has been shown in some clinical trials to improve walking distance by 40-50% [13, 14] after 3-6 months. However, in an analysis of several trials it only modestly improved walking distances; approximately 10 meters for the onset of pain and 20 meters for total walking distance [15]. People with heart failure should NOT take Pletal. Other additional medicines may serve to reduce your blood pressure, relax your blood vessels or reduce the work of your heart. The common (but not limited to) categories of these types of drugs are beta blockers, ACE inhibitors or calcium channel blockers. In addition to reduced blood flow, part of the disease process in PAD is the development of abnormal leg skeletal muscle. These abnormalities make a muscle very inefficient at utilizing oxygen. Two drugs that may help with this are L-carnitine and propionyl-L-carnitine. These drugs can improve a PAD patient's ability to walk by 50% [16]. Last, some of the most exciting new research is being conducted on drugs that are injected with a needle directly into muscle, called angiogenic growth factors (see below). These drugs show promise by initiating the growth of new blood vessels (angiogenesis). These have not been approved by the FDA and can only be obtained by entering a research clinical trial.

Therapeutic Angiogenesis: A Promising New Frontier in PAD Treatment

As described in this book, standard treatment for PAD includes risk factor modification (blood pressure, cholesterol, weight control), exercise training, smoking cessation and making sure you are on the proper medications. If these do not successfully improve a patient's condition, surgical revascularization in the form of angioplasty, stents, or vein bypass grafting may be necessary. However, in some cases none of these treatments relieve the symptom of claudication or decrease the progression of disease. These patients may be candidates for a new treatment called therapeutic angiogenesis. Simply put, therapeutic angiogenesis refers to an emerging field in medicine that infuses a drug into the artery or injects a drug into muscles that are not receiving enough blood in order to grow new blood vessels. Potential patients who may benefit from this new therapy include those who have had several failed surgeries, have blockages that are not in an area that is operable or those who have critical limb ischemia (pain at rest).

To date, there have been few human clinical trials performed on therapeutic angiogenesis. However, the results of the few that have been reported are very promising. In one study done at the National Institutes of Health (NIH) [17], PAD patients with claudication and an ABI of less than 0.80 were given this treatment. The drugs improved calf blood flow after 1 month and 6 months of treatment. In a larger trial [18] PAD patients improved their walking times after 3 months of treatment. A third trial [19] did not show an improvement over a placebo. Based on these studies, it is clear that therapeutic angiogenesis will eventually become accepted as a treatment option in some cases. But, until the medical community discovers the best way to deliver these vessel sprouting drugs, this option will only be available through research clinical trials.

> **The most important thing to remember from this chapter:** There is strong clinical evidence that drug therapy can reduce death, slow progression of vascular disease and help you be able to walk longer without leg pain. It is likely your doctor will prescribe a combination of drugs that includes: statins or other cholesterol reducing medications, antiplatelets, blood pressure medicine, ACE inhibitors or beta blockers. It is important to understand why you are taking each and know the potential contraindications specific to your situation.

References

1) LaRosa JC, He J, Vupputuri S. Effects of statins on risk of coronary disease. A meta-analysis of randomized controlled trials. JAMA 1999; 282:2340-2346.
2) Pignone M, Phillips C, Mulrow C. Use of lipid lowering drugs for primary prevention of coronary heart disease: meta-analysis of randomized trials. BMJ 2000; 321(7267):983-6.
3) Furberg CD. Effects of pravastatin on coronary disease events in sub-groups defined by coronary risk factors. Circulation. 2000; 102:1893-2000.321:1-5.
4) Heart Protection Study Group. MRC/BHF Heart Protection Study of cholesterol lowering with simvastatin in 20,535 high risk individuals: a randomized placebo controlled trial. Lancet. 2002; 360:7-22.
5) Mondillo S, Ballo P, Barbati R, Guerrini F, Ammaturo T, Agricola E, Pastore M, Borrello F, Belcastro M, Picchi A, Nami R. Effects of simvistatin on walking performance and symptoms of intermittent claudication in hypercholesteremic patients with peripheral vascular disease. Am J Med. 2003; 114:359-364.
6) Pedersen TR, Kjekshus J, Pyorala K. Effect of simvstatin on ischemic signs and symptoms in the Scandinavian simvastatin survival study(4S). Am. J. Card. 1998; 81:333.

7) Mohler ER, Hiatt WR, Creager MA. Cholesterol reduction with atorvastatin improves walking distance in patients with peripheral arterial disease. Circulation. 2003; 108:1481.

8) Antithrombitic Trialist' Collaboration: Collaborative meta-analysis of randomized trials of antiplatelet therapy for prevention of death, myocardial infarction, and stroke in high risk patients. BMJ. 2002; 1994; 324:71-76.

9) CAPRIE Steering Committee. A randomised, blinded, trial of clopidogrel versus aspirin in patients at risk of ischaemic events (CAPRIE). Lancet. 1996;348:1329-1339.

10) Clopidogrel in Unstable Angina to Prevent Recurrent Events (CURE) Trial Investigators. Effects of clopidogrel in addition to aspirin in patients with acute coronary syndromes without ST-segment elevation. NEJM. 2001; 345(23):494–502.

11) Girolami B, Bernardi E, Prins MH. Treatment of intermittent claudication with physical training, smoking cessation, pentoxifyline or nafronyl: a meta-anlaysis. Arch Intern Med. 1999; 159:337-345.

12) Porter JM, Cutler BS, Lee BY, Reich T, Reichle FA, Scogin JT, Strandness DE. Pentoxifylline efficacy in the treatment of intermittent claudication: multicenter controlled double-blind trial with objective assessment of chronic occlusive arterial disease patients. Am Heart J. 1982;104(1):66-72.

13) Dawson DL, Cutler BS, Meissner MH, Strandness DE Jr. Cilostrazol has beneficial effects in the treatment of intermittent claudication. Circulation 1998; 98:678-686.

14) Money SR, Herd JA, Isaacson JL. Effect of cilostazol on walking distances with intermittent claudication caused by peripheral vascular disease. J Vasc Surg. 1998; 27:267-274.

15) Bedenis R, Stewart M, Cleanthis M, Robless P, Mikhailidis DP, Stansby G. Cilostazol for intermittent claudication. Cochrane Database Syst Rev. 2014;10:CD003748.

16) Hiatt WR, Regensteiner JG, Creager MA, Hirsch AT, Cooke JP, Olin JW, Gorbunov GN, Isner J, Lukjanov YV, Tsitsiashvili MS, Zabelskaya TF, Amato A. Propionyl-L-carnitine improves exercise performance and functional status in patients with claudication. Am J Med. 2001;110(8):616-22.

17) Lazarous DF, Unger EF, Epstein SE, Stine A, Arevalo JL, Chew EW, Quyyumi AA. Basic fibroblast growth factor in patients with intermittent claudication: Results of a phase I trial. J Am Coll Cardiol. 2000; 36:1239-1244.

18) Lederman RG, Mendelsohn FO, Anderson RD, Saucedo JS, Tenaglia AN, Hermiller JB, Hillegas WB, Rocha-Singh K, Moon TE, Whitehouse MJ, Annex BH; TRAFFIC Investigators. Therapeutic angiogenesis with recombinant fibroblast growth factor-2 for intermittent claudication (the TRAFFIC study): A randomized trial. Lancet 2002; 359:2053-2058.

19) Rajagopolan S, Mohler ER, Lederman RJ, Mendelsohn FO, Saucedo JF, Goldman CK, Blebea J, Macko J, Kessler PD, Rasmussen HS, Annex BH. Regional angiogenesis with vascular endothelial growth factor in peripheral arterial disease. A Phase II, randomized, double-blind controlled study of adenoviral delivery of vascular endothelial growth factor-121 in patients with disabling intermittent claudication. Circulation 2003; 108:1933-1938.

Chapter 9

The Relationship between Type 2 Diabetes and PAD

Type 2 diabetes accounts for approximately 90% of diabetes, with the other 10% due to type1 and gestational diabetes. This chapter will focus on type 2 diabetes. Type 2 Diabetes is a cause of major health concern and its prevalence is rising largely due to an increase in obesity and sedentary lifestyles. Patients with diabetes live 5-10 years less than non-diabetics, mainly due to accelerated and more severe atherosclerosis. The prevalence of diagnosed diabetes is 13.9 million people in the U.S., with an equal amount having undiagnosed diabetes. According to the American Diabetes Association, the estimated prevalence of diabetes in the U.S. was 7.4% in 1995, and expected to be 9% by 2025. Therefore, if you have PAD and other risk factors such as being overweight and sedentary, you should ask your doctor to test for diabetes. **You may have diabetes and not know it! Therefore, if you have been diagnosed with PAD, ask your doctor to check your fasting sugar levels for diabetes.**

> **Approximately 20% of all PAD patients also have diabetes.**

Since 1990, the prevalence has increased by 61% in the U.S.! The worldwide prevalence of diabetes is projected to rise from 171 million in 2000, to 300 million in 2010 and 366 million in 2030! It affects non-Caucasians more than Caucasians and women more than men. It contributes to heart disease, kidney failure and blindness. <u>**Along with smoking, diabetes is the greatest risk factor for PAD,**</u> including the most advanced and severe type of PAD, critical limb ischemia. It is easy to point out the seriousness of diabetes in PAD. To put it simply, individuals with diabetes are more likely to have PAD and have an accelerated progression of PAD. Approximately 65% of people with diabetes will die of heart disease or stroke. PAD patients who also have diabetes have more extensive and severe PAD and have a greater chance of vessel calcification [1]. The severity of PAD in those with diabetes is more, as large blood vessels are affected earlier in the disease and small blood vessels tend to be more affected than in those without diabetes. Among PAD patients who are also diabetic, gangrene develops in approximately 1/3 compared to only 5% who are non-diabetic

PAD patients. The combination of PAD and diabetes means a 2-4 fold risk of intermittent claudication and a 10-16 fold increase in amputation [2]. In the Framingham Study, 20 out of 100 patients with claudication had diabetes versus only 6 out of 100 without claudication. In addition, almost 4 in 10 diabetic PAD patients have pain at rest (critical limb ischemia) and 50% will die after only 5 years [3]. In addition to complicating PAD, other health concerns to consider are that every year 24,000 people in the U.S. go blind because of diabetes and people over 65 years old are twice as likely to be hospitalized for kidney infections as patients without diabetes.

Of those people with high blood glucose, approximately 30-50% will go on to develop diabetes within 5 years.

What is Diabetes and How is it Diagnosed? Diabetes is one of the oldest diseases known to man, and remains one of our nation's top 10 killers. First described in 400 B.C., the Greek word diabetes translates to "run through a siphon" and the Latin word mellitus translates to "honey." Diabetes simply means you have too much sugar (glucose) in your blood. Under normal conditions, your pancreas secretes insulin, which then circulates in the bloodstream and allows glucose to enter cells to use as energy. As blood glucose levels drop, so does the amount of insulin secreted; thereby maintaining a balance of insulin and glucose to keep blood glucose levels normal. In type 2 diabetes, there is a combination of insufficient insulin production from pancreas and the inability of cells to respond adequately to normal levels of insulin; a term called insulin resistance. Insulin resistance occurs primarily within the muscles, liver, and fat tissue. The result is a build-up of glucose in your bloodstream. The hallmark symptoms of diabetes include fatigue, weakness, constant hunger, excessive thirst and frequent urination. Diabetes can be diagnosed by your doctor by either a blood test or a urine test. Your doctor will look for elevated levels of sugar in your blood or urine or elevated acetone (ketones) in your urine. **<u>Diabetes is defined by a fasting blood glucose value of greater than 125 mg/ dL in the blood.</u>** The table above illustrates a range for normal and diabetic fasting blood glucose values.

Blood Glucose Concentration

Normal Blood Glucose Values (mg/dl)	
Fasting	65 to 100
Two Hours After a Meal	100 to 125
Pre-Diabetic (Impaired) Values	
Fasting	100 to 125
Two Hours After a Meal	125 to 150
Diabetes Mellitis Values	
Fasting	higher than 125
Two Hours After a Meal	higher than 180

Your doctor may also order a blood test for Glycated/Glycosylated Hemoglobin A1c. What is this? It measures the percentage of blood sugar attached to hemoglobin, the oxygen-carrying protein in red blood cells. Glycosylated Hemoglobin or Hemoglobin A1c represents your "average" levels of glucose over the past 8 to 12 weeks. This provides an additional criterion for assessing glucose control because glycated hemoglobin values are free of day-to-day glucose fluctuations and are unaffected by recent exercise or recent food ingestion. **Normal values of Hemoglobin A1c are 5.7%-6.4%. An A1C level of 6.5 percent or higher on two separate tests indicates that you have diabetes.** Glycosylated Hemoglobin should be routinely monitored by your doctor every 3-4 months.

Due to the increased risk when both PAD and diabetes are present, patients should practice aggressive blood glucose control. PAD patients with diabetes should check their fasting blood glucose every morning, talk to their doctors about medications, maintain an ideal weight and exercise. If values are consistently out of range, you should contact your doctor.

> If you have diabetes and any of the following occurs, you should seek medical attention because it is an indication your ketones are dangerously high:
> - Feeling dazed and confused
> - A "fruity" smell to your breath
> - A blood glucose reading of greater than 300 mg/dl
> - A feeling of nausea with flushed skin

What is the Link between Diabetes and PAD?

There is no question that elevated blood glucose is related to the development of PAD. One study has shown that as little as a 1% increase in HbA1c was associated with a 28% increase in risk of PAD [4]! In addition, this study suggested that the length of time a patient had diabetes was also related to increased PAD risk. However, little is known about the unique biology that occurs with the combination of PAD and diabetes. We do know that diabetics are at very high risk for developing PAD or a higher rate of progression of already existing PAD because of its negative affect on the function of blood vessel walls, the blood flow and cholesterol levels. PAD patients with diabetes have similar blockages in arteries above and surrounding the knee (femoral artery) as those without diabetes, but have more diffuse distal disease in the arteries below the joint (e.g. tibial, infrapopliteal and peroneal arteries), and more nerve damage than PAD patients without diabetes [5]. Distal disease involves blockages in the narrow part of an artery or in areas branching out from a main artery. Unfortunately, severe distal disease often results in less successful surgical revascularization. Diabetes causes premature aging to the cells that line blood vessel walls, increases fatty deposits on arterial walls and promotes increased synthesis of triglycerides and bad cholesterol in the liver. Diabetes has a negative effect on the coaguability ("stickiness") of blood by causing cells (platelets) to clump together. In addition, the blood vessels of diabetic patients do not expand (dilate) and contract (constrict) normally. Diabetic PAD patients are far less likely to sprout collateral blood vessels than non-diabetic. All of the above decreases blood flow and starves the muscles of oxygen. If untreated, nerve damage may occur and prevent a patient from feeling the hallmark warning sign of PAD, such as claudication, or cause a foot injury to go unnoticed. Having diabetes increases the likelihood of coronary atherosclerosis by 400% [6]! **<u>The combination of diabetes and PAD causes poor blood supply to your feet, damages the nerves that tell you your feet are hurting and reduces your ability to fight infection. All of these reasons are why diabetes is the most common cause of amputation in the United States,</u>** accounting for 45% to 70% of all non-accident related amputations [7]. PAD patients with diabetes have a 12 fold increase in amputation risk compared to non-diabetic PAD patients [8]. In patients age 65 to 74, diabetes increases the risk for amputation by 20 fold [8]! Even the most minor injury like a blister, cut or abrasion can lead to infection.

The effect diabetes has on walking ability in patients with PAD has not been well studied. Some studies suggest that PAD patients with diabetes are unable to walk as far as PAD alone, have poor balance and cannot walk as fast. This reduced ability to walk has been explained by diabetic neuropathy, differences in exertional leg symptoms, and greater cardiovascular disease.

PAD and Other Risk Factors

Diabetes by itself is a risk factor for coronary artery disease. Once diabetes begins to affect the body, other risk factors of atherosclerosis become more serious. For example, diabetic patients with high LDL cholesterol and high blood pressure are related to the development of PAD and more likely to have claudication.

> **The American Diabetes Association Consensus Statement on PAD in those People with Diabetes.**
>
> **Due to the high estimated prevalence of PAD in patients with diabetes:**
>
> **A screening ABI should be performed in patients over 50 years old who have known diabetes. If normal, the test should be repeated every 5 years.**
>
> **A screening ABI should be considered in diabetic patients under 50 years old if they have other known atherosclerosis risk factors (smoking, hypertension, poor cholesterol or diabetes for less than 10 years).**

PAD Diabetics with Hypertension

Not only is hypertension a risk factor for PAD by itself, but also is an additional concern for those PAD patients with diabetes. **It is reported that each 10 mm Hg rise in systolic blood pressure is associated with a 25% risk for PAD**. Furthermore, a 10 mm Hg reduction in systolic blood pressure reduces the risk for limb amputation by 16%. Other studies have shown blood pressure control with medications significantly reduced the risk of a cardiovascular event or completely eliminated the risk of a cardiovascular event related to PAD [9]. The American Diabetes Association has advised that patients with both PAD and diabetes maintain resting blood pressures below 130/80 mm Hg for the purpose of decreasing cardiovascular risk [10].

PAD Diabetics with Bad Cholesterol

As stated earlier, there is bad cholesterol (LDL's), good cholesterol (HDL's) and total cholesterol. Interestingly, the total cholesterol values in diabetics do not appear to be much different than people without diabetes. However, type 2 diabetics have higher small dense LDL particles and lower HDL levels compared to non-diabetics. Low levels of HDL have recently been identified as an independent risk factor for patients with PAD [11]. Previously, the National Cholesterol Education Program/Adult Treatment Panel III identified diabetes as an independent risk factor for coronary artery disease and recommended that LDL be reduced to less than 70 in patients who have both PAD and diabetes [12]. More recently, guidelines for cholesterol have been further updated. These recommendations, discussed in detail in chapter 5, state PAD patients with diabetes should be on moderate to high doses of statin drugs. Furthermore, based on recommendations of the Inter-Society Consensus for the Management of Peripheral Arterial Disease it is recommended a LDL goal of < 100 mg/dL in patients with PAD; preferentially by using statin drugs. In higher risk PAD patients, a goal of < 70 mg/dL is recommended (6,13). Statins, a common medication used for patients with poor cholesterol values, have been shown to be helpful in preventing PAD surgeries, angioplasty, and amputation in diabetics [14].

Management of Diabetes

Diabetes is not curable and requires constant attention for a lifetime. The PAD patient with diabetes is at increased risk due to the combination of risk factors shared by diabetes and atherosclerosis. All risk factors that are modifiable by lifestyle (e.g. smoking and diet) or medication (e.g. blood pressure and cholesterol) should be taken very seriously and recommendations from your doctor adhered to. The goal is to maintain normal blood glucose levels and prevent additional complications. The American Diabetic Association has identified three essential components to managing diabetes. They are diet, exercise and medication.

> **MYTH: Diabetics should avoid foods high in sugar (e.g. candy). Currently, science does not support this commonly thought of rule. Rather than depriving yourself of sweet treats, consider only moderate amounts and eating a mixture of protein and fat along with carbohydrates to maintain your blood sugar level.**

Diet. Contrary to popular belief, there is no proven diet specific for diabetes. According to the American Diabetes Association, there is no standard meal plan or eating pattern that works universally for all people with diabetes (15). In order to be effective, nutrition and eating habits should be individualized for each patient. It is safe to say that diabetics should focus on eating a healthy nutrient dense diet with minimal processed foods. By eating well balanced, properly timed and portioned meals many diabetics can control their disease through diet alone. Eating a proper diet can prevent weight gain (a major risk factor for insulin abnormalities), control blood pressure, lower cholesterol and maintain blood glucose levels. If you have diabetes, we highly recommend meeting with a nutritionist for additional tips on how to meal plan and cook. All dieticians have helpful hand-out information that will tell you how to modify your diet based your personal goals and preferences.

Exercise. The known benefits of exercise for diabetic patients are a decrease in blood glucose and improved insulin action. Before starting an exercise program, it is recommended to seek consult with your physician, and if possible, an exercise physiologist. Some considerations include when to exercise relative to insulin levels or your medications, when to snack and what type of food to eat before and after exercise, and how often to check your blood glucose levels. Regular exercise will also improve other risk factors for PAD such as lowering blood pressure, increasing HDL (good cholesterol), help maintain proper weight and positively affect skeletal muscle's ability to handle glucose.

Medications and Clinical Trials. Clinical trials evaluating glucose control have shown promise by a trend toward a reduction in peripheral vascular events, but unfortunately have not been statistically significant. For example, the Diabetes Control and Complications Trial reported a 22% relative risk decrease in lower limb problems and a 42% reduction when combining coronary and peripheral problems [16]. Another trial, The UK Prospective Diabetes Study (UKPDS), demonstrated a trend toward lower death rates from PAD and less amputations with tight blood glucose control (17). Other Recent studies show that patients with both diabetes and PAD benefit greatly from medications used to treat hypertension and elevated triglycerides with low HDL. Statin therapy has reduced the number of cardiovascular events in PAD diabetics with coronary artery disease and high LDL cholesterol by 55%. Last, clinical trials indicate all PAD diabetics should be on antiplatelet medication unless there is a contraindication [18].

PAD and Foot Care. Diabetes poses an additional threat to the feet of PAD patients due to the lack of circulation, potential nerve damage, increased wound healing time and chance of infection. Therefore, it is important that you take precaution not to put your feet at increased risk for injury. Below is a list of common practices all PAD patients with diabetes should be in the habit of performing.

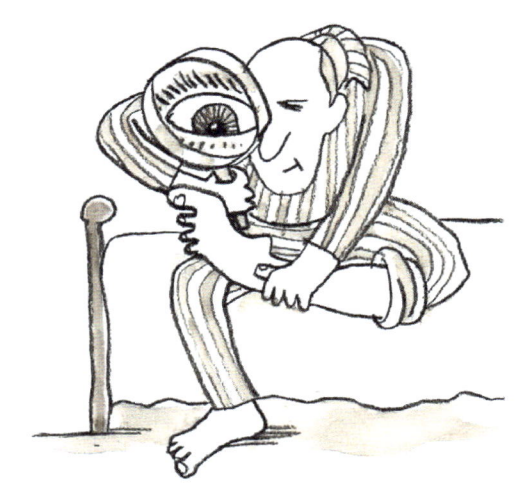

> **DO's and DON'Ts of Foot Care for Patients with PAD and Diabetes**
>
> - **Do check your feet every day for sores, cuts, blisters, etc.**
> - **Do practice good foot hygiene by cleaning daily and changing your socks**
> - **Do keep your feet warm to improve circulation**
> - **Do NOT choose shoes that are too tight or cause friction that may lead to blisters**
> - **Do NOT walk around barefoot**
> - **Do NOT treat corns, ingrown toenails, calluses, etc. yourself. Call your doctor for help if these common foot ailments need treatment.**

Because of the added risk to PAD patients it is recommended to have an annual check-up with your doctor that includes the following tests:

- Blood glucose/hemoglobin A1C
- Blood lipids (cholesterol)
- Foot exam
- Kidney function
- Eye exam
- Blood pressure

> **The most important thing to remember from this chapter:** Diabetes is caused by your body's inability to use insulin and utilize sugar as a fuel. This causes excess sugar in your bloodstream. Normal fasting blood glucose values should be 70-100 mg/dL. Higher blood glucose concentrations cause damage to artery walls. Because PAD patients are already at risk due to poor circulation, this added burden increases amputation, nerve damage and wound healing. Diabetes should be controlled by diet, exercise and medication. All diabetic PAD patients should have their blood glucose checked regularly because you may have high blood sugar and not know it!

References
1) Beckman JA, Craeger MA, Libby P. Diabetes and atherosclerosis: Epidemiology, pathophysiology and management. JAMA. 2002; 287:2570.
2) Uusitupa M, Niskanen L, Siitonen O, Pyorala K. 5 year incidence of atherosclerotic vascular disease in relation to gender, risk factors, insulin level and abnormalities in lipoproteins in non-insulin dependent diabetics and non-diabetic individuals. Circulation 1990; 82:27-36.
3) Reiber Ge, Pecoraro RE, Koepsell TD. Risk factors for amputation in patients with diabetes mellitus. A case-control study. Ann Intern Med. 1992; 117:97-105.
4) Adler A, Stevens R, Neil A, Stratton I, Boulton A, Holman R. UKPDS: Hyperglycaemia and other potentially modifiable risk factors for peripheral arterial disease in type 2 diabetes. Diabetes Care 2002; 25:894-899.

5) Jude EB, Oyibo SO, Chalmers N, Boulton AJ. Peripheral arterial disease in diabetic and nondiabetic patients: A comparison of severity and outcomes. Diabetes Care. 2001; 14:1433.

6) Norgren L, Hiatt WR, Dormandy JA, Nehler MR, Harris KA, Fowkes FGR;TASC II Working Group. Inter-Society Consensus for the Management of Peripheral Arterial Disease (TASC II). J Vasc Vasc Surg. 2007; 45(S1): S5-S67.

7) Faxon DP, et al Atherosclerotic Vascular Disease Conference Writing Group III: Pathophysiology. Circulation. 2004; 109:2617-2625.

8) MMWR Morb Mortal Wkly Rep. Diabetes-related amputations of lower extremities in the medicare population Minnesota, 1933-1995. 1998; 47:649-652.

9) Mehler PS, Coll JR, Estacio R, Esler A, Schrier RW, Hiatt WR. Intensive blood pressure control reduces the risk of cardiovascular events in patients with peripheral arterial disease and type 2 diabetes. Circulation 2003; 107:753-756.

10) Collins R, Armitage J, Parish S, Sleight P, Peto R. MRC/BHF Heart Protection Study of cholesterol lowering with with simvastatin in 5963 people with diabetes: a randomized placebo controlled trial. Lancet 2003; 361:2005-2016.

11) Adler A, Stevens R, Neil A, Stratton I, Boulton A, Holman R. UKPDS: Hyperglycaemia and other potentially modifiable risk factors for peripheral arterial disease in type 2 diabetes. Diabetes Care 2002; 25:894-899.

12) Grundy SM, Cleeman JI, Bairey Merz CN. Implications of recent clinical trials for the National Cholesterol Education Program Adult Treatment Panel III Guidelines. J Am Coll Cardiol. 2004; 44:720-732.

13) Pollak AW, Kramer CM. LDL lowering in peripheral arterial disease. Are there benefits beyond reducing cardiovascular morbidity and mortality? Clin Lipidology 2012; 7(2):141-149.

14) Collins R, Armitage J, Parish S, Sleight P, Peto R. MRC/BHF Heart Protection Study of cholesterol lowering with with simvastatin in 5963 people with diabetes: a randomized placebo controlled trial. Lancet 2003; 361:2005-2016.

15) Evert AB, Boucher JL, Cypress M, Dunbar SA, Franz MJ, Mayer-Davis EJ, Neumiller JJ, Nwankwo R, Verdi CL, Urbanski P, Yancy WS Jr. Nutrition therapy recommendations for the management of adults with diabetes. Diabetes Care. 2014;37 Suppl 1:S120-43.

16) DCCT Study Group. Effect of intense diabetes management on macrovasculature events and risk factors in the Diabetes Control and Complications Trial. Am J Card. 1995; 894-903.

17) UK Prospective Diabetes Study (UKPDS) Group. Intensive blood glucose control with sulphonylureas or insulin compared with conventional treatment and risk of complication in patients with type 2 diabetes (UKPDS 33). Lancet 1998;352(9131):837-53.
18) ACC/AHA 2005 guidelines for the management of patients with peripheral artery disease: Executive Summary. Journal of the Amer Coll Cardiol. 2006; 47(6):1239-1312.

Chapter 10
What is a Revascularization?

The term **"revascularization,"** or sometimes called an "intervention" usually refers to either angioplasty (endovascular) or bypass graft surgery (open) in order to improve blood supply to your lower extremity. These procedures are considered when optimal drug therapy, exercise and risk factor modification by healthy lifestyle (e.g. smoking cessation) do not improve your symptoms (leg pain) or ability to walk. If you are a candidate for revascularization, your doctor will likely perform "imaging studies" to better understand your anatomy and the severity of your disease. These imaging studies (e.g. angiography, ultrasound, MRI) have been described in chapter 2. Once this has been done, a decision on angioplasty/stent or open surgical bypass will be made with you. When making this decision, important things to consider are risk/benefits, your expectations, and the durability of the revascularization. Durability refers to the likelihood that your artery will remain open after a certain time period, usually 1-5 years.

Endovascular Percutaneous Transluminal Angioplasty (PTA) and Stenting

The aim of this procedure is to stretch open a segment of a narrowed or blocked artery using a balloon. To do this a small needle (catheter), with a balloon on the tip, is inserted to the point where the blockage is occurring. This procedure is done in a catheterization laboratory and usually takes between 1-2 hours from start to finish. On the day of your procedure, small electrodes will be placed on your chest to monitor your heart. After injection of local anesthetic, a sheath is inserted and guided into the leg artery where the blockage is located. Once the site has been identified, the doctor inserts the small catheter with a tiny deflated balloon at the tip.

Balloon Angioplasty

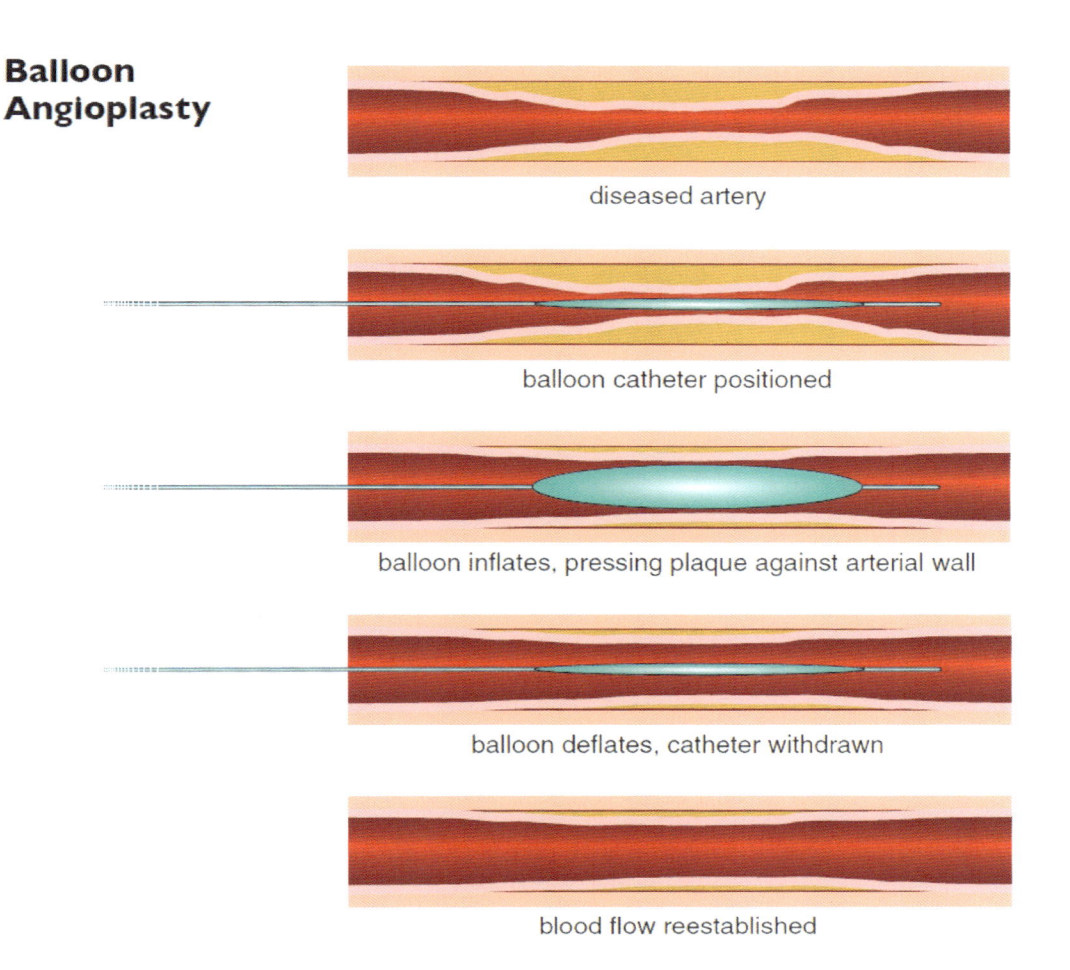

diseased artery

balloon catheter positioned

balloon inflates, pressing plaque against arterial wall

balloon deflates, catheter withdrawn

blood flow reestablished

This is done by watching a monitor and guiding the balloon into the exact area of blockage. A contrast agent, or dye, is injected into the catheter, producing an X-ray image that appears on a special screen. This helps the doctor pinpoint the location of the blockage. The balloon is then repeatedly inflated to push the plaque against the artery wall, thereby widening the artery. Angioplasty is a relatively safe procedure with similar complication as an arteriogram. It is common to have some pain and bruising at the site of the insertion on your thigh. The risk of death is about 1 in 1,000. You will likely remain in the hospital for 24 hours and be able to go home the following day.

Artery before and after balloon angioplasty.

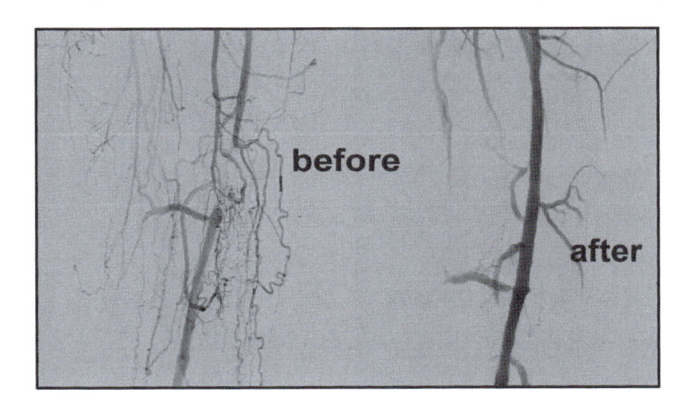

A stent can be put in during this procedure. A stent is a wire mesh tube that is permanently inserted into an artery at the site of blockage to help keep it from closing up again. The stent works by acting as a scaffold to provide support inside the artery.

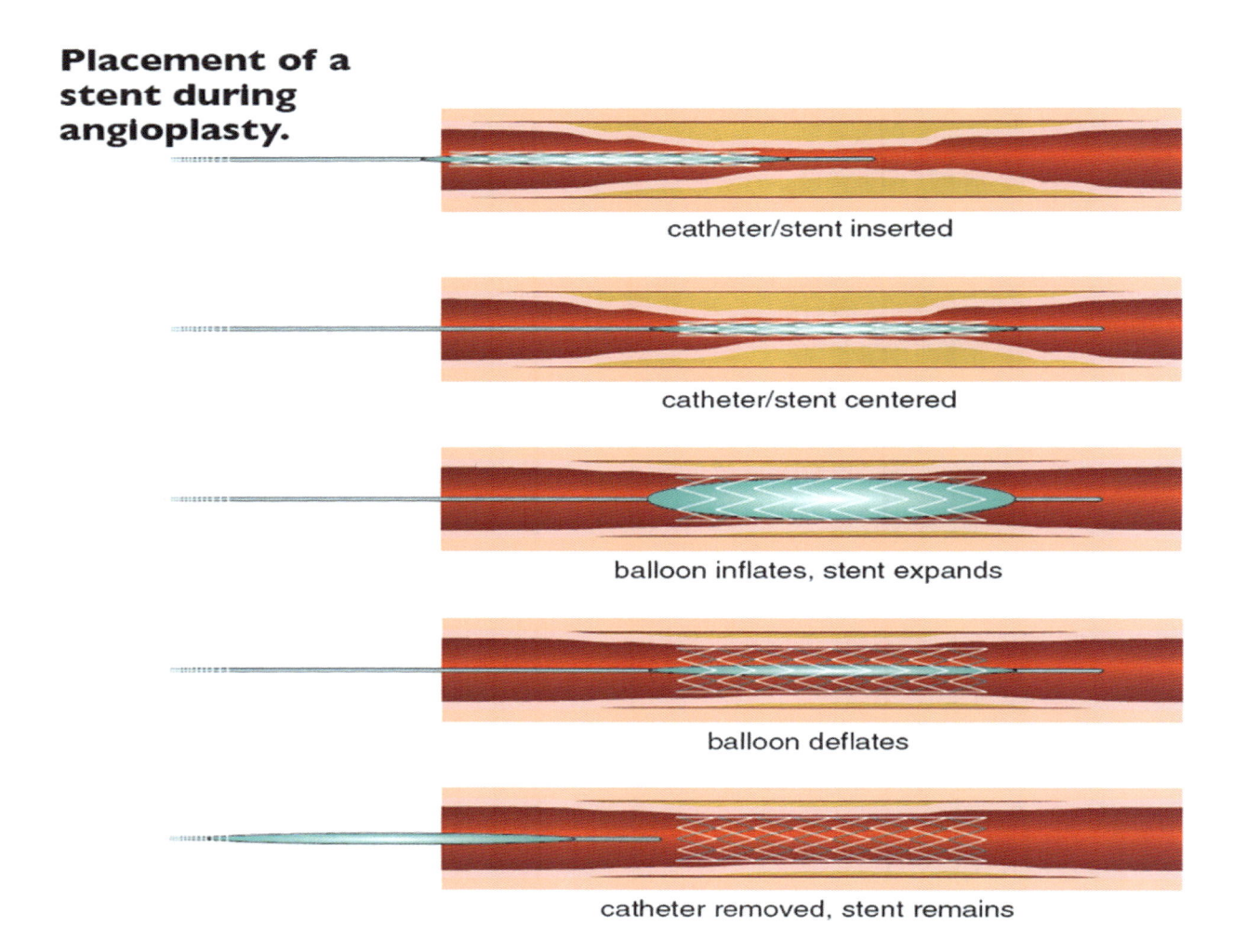

Placement of a stent during angioplasty.

catheter/stent inserted

catheter/stent centered

balloon inflates, stent expands

balloon deflates

catheter removed, stent remains

The majority of patients enjoy immediate relief of symptoms after angioplasty in terms of walking performance. However, 5%-20% of cases are unsuccessful due to technical difficulties [1,2]. In addition, up to approximately 10% are technically successful, but do not improve symptoms. The following table lists potential reasons for unsuccessful interventions. Compared to bypass surgery, angioplasty is favorable because it is associated with lower morbidity (sickness and complications), requires only a short hospital stay and has a faster healing time than bypass surgery.

Picture of a stent

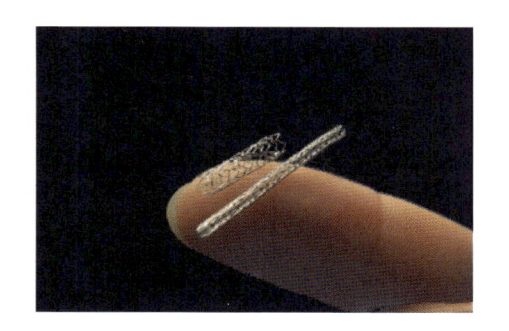

Problem	Reason for Potential Increased Risk or Complication
Long or diffuse disease	Require multiple stents, higher re-stenosis rates, time consuming and costly to treat
Heavy calcification	Resistant to mechanical approaches and may involve presence of diabetes
Multi-level disease (e.g. thigh and calf)	Often requires femoro-popliteal and infra-popliteal treatment simultaneously
Adductor canal disease	Treatment option minimal due to high range of motion in this area
Common femoral disease	Stenting increases risk to other arteries (profunda artery)

The TransAtlantic Inter-Society Consensus (TASC)

TASC has defined lesions (blockages) into 4 categories: Types A, B, C and D [3]. ***Why is this classification system important? It is important because, along with your symptoms, it will play a very important role on what type of treatment or revascularization procedure will be performed on you; either exercise, angioplasty/stent or surgical bypass.*** For example, type A lesions are the least complicated and should be treated with an endovascular approach (PTA); usually having excellent results. Type B lesions also have excellent results with endovascular interventions. Surgical revascularization (bypass) is recommended for type C lesions and is preferred over endovascular intervention unless there is a high risk for an open procedure. High risk may include smoking or diabetes. Type D lesions are most likely treated by a surgical approach. Further categorization is included in the tables below. The following tables in this chapter are given in great detail to describe lesion types (more than you likely need or want!) and should be discussed with your doctor. Your doctor can show you on an anatomy chart exactly what artery your lesion is located in and describe the severity. Based on the lesion location and severity, your doctor will likely follow the guidelines in these tables to help him/her decide what the best intervention is for you. Last, patency (success artery of being open) rates are also given. Below is a diagram showing the arteries of the lower leg. This will help you visualize where each artery is while reading these chapters.

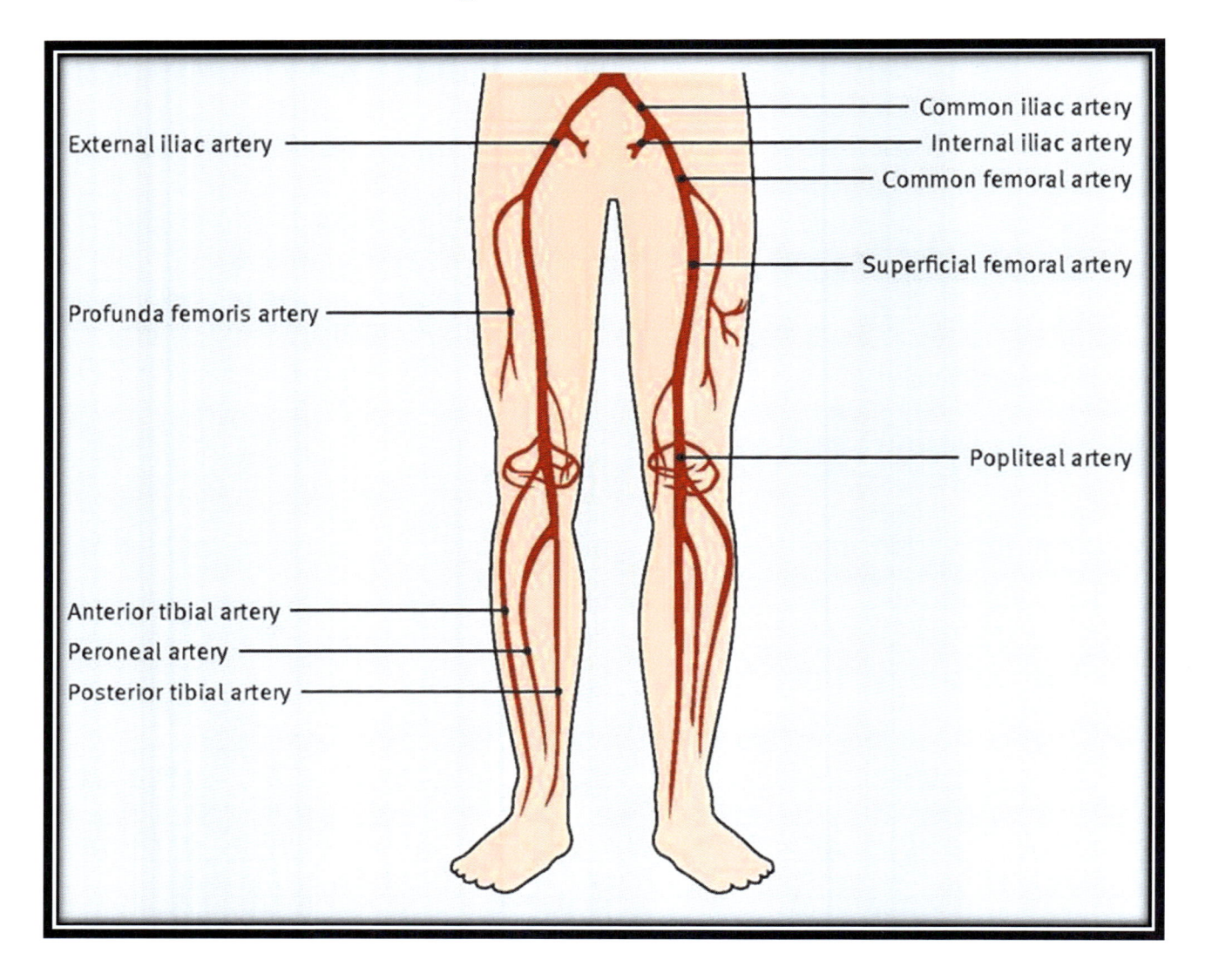

Arteries of the Lower leg

Abbreviations in the classification tables are as follows:

CFA- Common Femoral Artery
CIA- Common Iliac Artery
EIA- External Iliac Artery

Note: A stenosis is a blockage of 50%-95% and an occlusion is a blockage of 95%-100%.

Classification of Aorto-Iliac Lesions

Type A
Unilateral or Bilateral Stenoses of CIA
Unilateral or bilateral single short (≤ 3 cm) stenosis of EIA
Type B
Short (≤ 3 cm) stenosis of infra-renal aorta
Unilateral CIA occlusion
Single or multiple stenosis totaling 3-10 cm involving the EIA not extending into the CFA
Unilateral EIA occlusion not involving the origins of internal iliac or CFA
Type C
Bilateral CIA occlusions
Bilateral EIA stenoses 3-10 cm long not extending into the CFA
Unilateral EIA stenosis extending into the CFA
Unilateral EIA occlusion that involves the origins of internal iliac and/or CFA
Heavily calcified unilateral EIA occlusion with or without involvement of origins of internal iliac and/or CFA
Type D
Infra-renal aorto-iliac occlusion
Diffuse disease involving the aorta and both iliac arteries requiring treatment
Diffuse multiple stenoses involving the unilateral CIA, EIA and CFA
Unilateral occlusions of both CIA and EIA
Bilateral occlusions of EIA
Iliac stenoses in patients with AAA requiring treatment and not amenable to endograft placement or other lesions requiring open aortic or iliac surgery

Classification of Femoro-Popliteal Lesions

Type A
Single stenosis ≤10 cm in length
Single occlusion ≤ 5 cm in length
Type B
Multiple lesions (stenoses or occlusions), each ≤ 5 cm
Single stenosis or occlusion ≤ 15 cm not involving the infra geniculate popliteal artery
Single or multiple lesions in the absence of continuous tibial vessels to improve inflow for a distal bypass
Heavily calcified occlusion ≤ 5 cm in length
Single popliteal stenosis
Type C
Multiple stenoses or occlusions totaling >15 cm with or without heavy calcification
Recurrent stenoses or occlusions that need treatment after two endovascular interventions
Type D
Chronic total occlusions of CFA or SFA (>20 cm, involving the popliteal artery)
Chronic total occlusion of popliteal artery and proximal trifurcation vessels

In general, the success rates of angioplasty are greatest for lesions of the common iliac artery (CIA) and worsen the farther down the leg the lesion is, with increasing lesion length, number of lesions, number of smaller blood vessels off the artery, renal failure, diabetes and smoking.

Aorto-Iliac Revascularization by Endovascular (angioplasty/stent) Treatment

If you are having an angioplasty on your aorto-iliac artery because it is stenosed (50-95% blocked), you should feel good in the fact that the technical success, meaning after the procedure the artery is improved to at least < 50% blockage, is greater than 90% (3). And, after 5 years, the artery remains open (patent) in approximately 70-75% of people (4,5). Furthermore, if a stent was used, the artery remained open 74% of the time 8 years later (6). The table below summarized what is currently believed to be the success rates of aorto-iliac angioplasty (3).

Success Rates of Aorto-Iliac Angioplasty

Blockage %	Technical Success Rate	1 Year Success Rate	3 Year Success Rate	5 Year Success Rate
76%	96%	86%	82%	71%

To Stent or Not to Stent the Aorto-Iliac Artery?

There are very few studies directly comparing angioplasty vs stent; especially when you consider different lesion types and different definitions of success in each study. One study showed similar results between the two approaches, with 2 year success rates of 93% for angioplasty and 96% for stenting (7). The 5 year follow-up results were also very similar at 82% versus 80% (8). A statistical analysis compared and summarized several studies together and found success rates for stents was better than angioplasty; 96% vs 91% (9). Four-year success rates are summarized in the tables to follow. These tables are broken down by type of blockage (stenosis; 50%-95% blockage vs occlusion; 95%-100% blockage) and severity of symptoms (intermittent claudication (less severe) and critical limb ischemia (more severe)). The conclusion from this was that risk of long-term failure was reduced after stent placement compared with angioplasty for endovascular interventions on the aorto-iliac artery. It is important to note that this analysis was done in 1997 and current technical improvements would likely result in better results. Last, some more recent evidence also suggest that revascularization with stenting are comparable to an open surgical bypass (10,11,12,13).

Four Year Comparisons for Angioplasty vs Stent in Aorto-Iliac Arteries with Stenoses

Procedure and Patient Type	4 Year Success Rate
Angioplasty in IC	65%
Stent in IC	77%
Angioplasty in CLI	53%
Stent in CLI	67%

Four Year Comparisons for Angioplasty vs Stent in Aorto-Iliac Arteries with Occlusions

Procedure and Patient Type	4 Year Success Rate
Angioplasty in IC	54%
Stent in IC	61%
Angioplasty in CLI	44%
Stent in CLI	53%

IC = Intermittent Claudication (Less severe disease)
CLI = Critical Limb Ischemia (Very severe disease)

Aorto-Iliac Revascularization by Surgical Bypass

There are certain situations where a bypass graft is indicated over an angioplasty/stent for blockages in the lower extremity. If your symptoms are severe, lifestyle management has failed and you are not suitable for angioplasty or continue to have pain after several angioplasties, then bypass surgery is appropriate. The bypass vein will usually come from your own leg vein (e.g. the long saphenous vein) or a synthetic (man-made) graft (e.g. Dacron). Very much like heart bypass surgery, this graft is sewn above and below the blocked area to redirect or "bypass" the blockage and restore blood flow. In order to decide whether or not this is needed, an evaluation by angiogram, CTA and/or MRI is recommended to detect how diffuse the lesions are, presence of an aneurysm and amount of calcification. For surgical procedures requiring bypass there can be numerous presenting abnormalities regarding what exact vessels are blocked. The most common are blockages of the infrarenal aorta and iliac vessels. Blockages in these arteries usually cause pain in the buttock and thigh areas. Correction of these symptoms requires aorto-bifemoral bypass. The range of scenarios and appropriate surgical bypass options are beyond the scope of this book and should be discussed with your surgeon. The surgery involves going around the area of blockage (bypass) with a new vein to achieve normal blood flow again. Recently, surgeons have been performing an increased number of aorto-iliac revascularizations by laparoscopy. This minimally invasive approach has lower mortality rates, shorter hospital stay, less post-operative pain and faster return to normal activities. Ask your doctor if this is appropriate for you. However, most surgical revascularizations are still done by an open procedure. If there are blockages spread out in multiple areas of the aorto-iliac artery, then revascularization by surgical bypass is recommended. If there is a complete blockage (occlusion) of both the common and external iliac arteries or of the external iliac artery alone, then surgical bypass is usually performed. In addition, your doctor's decision will depend on if the disease also extends into the femoral artery, just below the iliac artery. A stent cannot be placed in this area because it will be affected when you bend your hip/knee. If this is the case, it is common to take a "hybrid" approach. A hybrid approach will combine a procedure of endarterectomy (a technique where your surgeon makes an incision in the artery and removes the plaque contained in the artery's inner lining) of the femoral artery with a stent in the iliac artery. In general, surgical reconstruction by direct vein bypass or synthetic material bypass and potentially endarterectomy is recommended in the aorta-iliac if there is diffuse disease which cannot be resolved by angioplasty/stent, you have had previously failed angioplasty/stent procedures or in situation of combined 95%-100% blockages and aneurysmal disease (14). The most common bypass, from the aorta to both femoral arteries, has a 5 year success rate of approximately 85%-90% and 10 year success rate of approximately 70%-85% (14,15). There are several options on what type of bypass can be used that are beyond the scope and purpose of this book. The table below was adopted from the Society of Vascular Surgery. This table shows the 5 year success rates of different types of bypass surgeries and angioplasty for patients with intermittent claudication [14]. Needless to say, surgical revascularization is a serious and complicated procedure. This information is intended to only familiarize you with some of the terms and provide approximate success rates. It is recommended that you discuss your specific situation with your doctor for the best options.

5 Year Success Rates for Different Revascularization Procedures of the Aorto-Iliac Artery in Patients with Intermittent Claudication

Type of Revascularization	5 Year Success Rate
Angioplasty	63-79%
Aorto-Femoral Bypass	81-93%
Ilio-Femoral Bypass	73-88%
Femoro-Femoral Bypass	60-83%

Femoro-Popliteal Revascularization by Endovascular (angioplasty/stent) Treatment

Blockages in the femoro-popliteal artery usually cause intermittent claudication pain in the calf. Angioplasty/stent is the preferred treatment for intermittent claudication for lesions up to 10 cm in length in the femoro-popliteal artery (1,3,14). Due to the development of new devices and techniques, it is now possible to treat even more advance lesions by angioplasty/stent (16). An effort was made to summarize the results of endovascular angioplasty/stent in the femoro-popliteal artery (17). This summary is in the tables on the following pages. Observation from this summary tells us several things. First, patients with less severe disease (only a partial blockage and intermittent claudication symptoms) do better than those with complete blockages and more severe symptoms (critical limb ischemia). Second, it appears from this summary that stent placement has better success rates than balloon angioplasty alone regardless of disease severity.

The tables on the following tables show very high technical success rates. The first table demonstrates the results of a meta-analysis (statistical summary) study. The second table comes from the American Heart Association and American College of Cardiology [18]. These data further extend the predictability of a specific intervention across different arteries. There are subtle differences between these tables. This can likely be accounted for by factors previously mentioned, such as the length and number of lesions. Other factors include location of the lesion and health of the arteries above and below the lesion. In addition, the type of stent may also be a factor in success rates [19,20,21,22,23]. New treatment options for interventions in PAD are developing at a rapid pace. New techniques and improved stents are currently in clinical trials. For these reasons is important for your doctor to discuss the current options available to you.

Summary of Results for Angioplasty and Stent in the Femoro-Popliteal Artery of Intermittent Claudication (Less Severe Disease)

Partial Blockage (Stenosis) & Year	Angioplasty Success Rate	Stent Placement Success Rate
Technical Success	99%	99%
1	77%	75%
2	66%	67%
3	61%	66%
4	57%	-
5	55%	-
Complete Blockage (Occlusion) & Year	Angioplasty Success Rate	Stent Placement Success Rate
Technical Success	88%	99%
1	65%	73%
2	54%	66%
3	48%	64%
4	44%	-
5	42%	-

Summary of Results for Angioplasty and Stent in the Femoro-Popliteal Artery of Critical Limb Ischemia (More Severe Disease)

Partial Blockage (Stenosis) & Year	Angioplasty Success Rate	Stent Placement Success Rate
Technical Success	83%	99%
1	60%	74%
2	49%	66%
3	43%	65%
4	40%	-
5	38%	-
Complete Blockage (Occlusion) & Year	Angioplasty Success Rate	Stent Placement Success Rate
Technical Success	70%	98%
1	47%	73%
2	36%	65%
3	30%	63%
4	27%	-
5	25%	-

Success Rates for Femoro-Popliteal Disease and Infra-Popliteal Disease Stenoses in Patients with Claudication (From American Heart Association and the American College of Cardiology).

Artery & Procedure	Technical Success	1 Year	2 Year	3 Year	4 Year	5 Year
Iliac Angioplasty	96%	79%	72%	68%	65%	—
Iliac Stent	100%	91%	84%	80%	77%	—
Femoropopliteal Angioplasty	95%	79%	75%	74%	71%	68%
Femoropopliteal Stent	98%	62%	52%	43%	—	—
Infrapopliteal Angioplasty	93%	79%	74%	—	—	—

Comparing Revascularization of the Femoro-Popliteal: Angioplasty vs Surgical Bypass

Head to head comparisons of angioplasty vs surgical bypass for the femoro-popliteal artery are almost non-existent. This is because there are very clear guidelines that dictate the type of revascularization based on how extensive the disease and how long the lesion(s). Surgical bypass is used for extensive disease, long lesion(s) and severe symptoms (critical limb ischemia). Angioplasty is used for limited disease (e.g. one lesion), short lesion(s) and less severe symptoms (intermittent claudication).

The following figure summarizes 5 year success rates of angioplasty/stent versus surgical bypass. As discussed, success rates are dependent on the location (which artery) and the procedure performed. As you can see from the figure, in general the farther down the arterial tree, the lower the success rates. Also, in general, surgical bypass tends to a have a slightly higher success rate than angioplasty/stent.

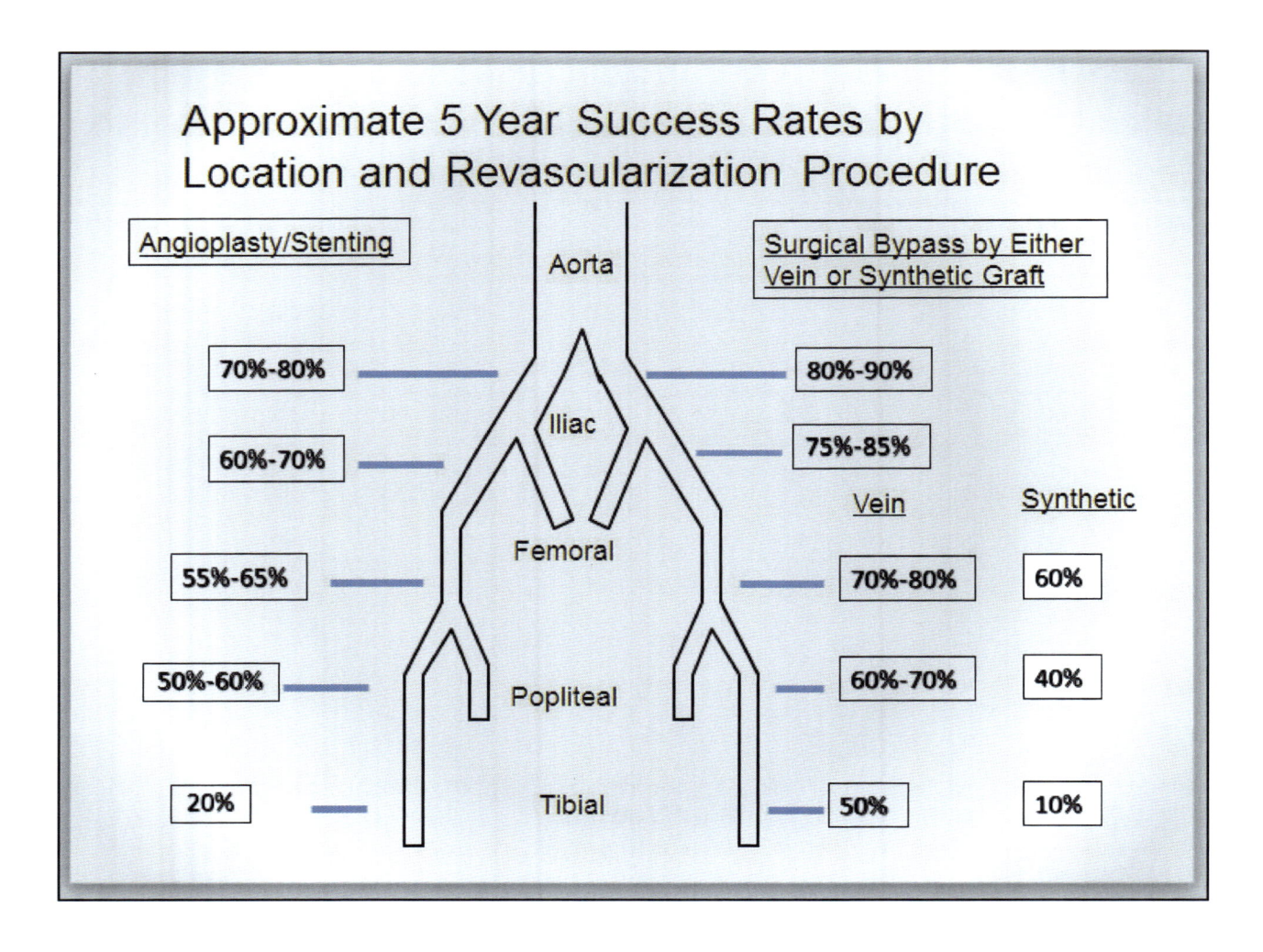

Approximate 5 Year Success Rates by Location and Revascularization Procedure

Angioplasty/Stenting	Location	Surgical Bypass by Either Vein or Synthetic Graft
	Aorta	
70%-80%	Iliac	80%-90%
60%-70%		75%-85%
		Vein / Synthetic
	Femoral	
55%-65%		70%-80% / 60%
50%-60%	Popliteal	60%-70% / 40%
20%	Tibial	50% / 10%

Recommendations for Revascularization

If you have read this far in this chapter, congratulations! As you can see, deciding on what type of revascularization is a case by case scenario and is complicated. The boxes on the pages to follow are some (but certainly not all) general recommendations adopted from the Society of Vascular Surgery [14] and the American Heart Association [24] for patients with intermittent claudication. Similar to the discussion in this chapter, the recommendation boxes are separated by type of artery, aorto-iliac and femoro-popliteal.

Recommendations for Aorto-Iliac Disease Revascularization

- Angioplasty/stent is favored over surgical bypass for less severe localized blockages (e.g. Type A lesion angioplasty/stent should be considered first for common iliac or external iliac disease).

- The use of bare metal or covered (ask your doctor about these) stents is recommended for the common iliac or external iliac disease.
- Covered stents are recommended if severe calcification or aneurysmal changes are present if there is a risk of rupture.
- In cases of severe disease, either angioplasty/stent or surgical bypass may be appropriate, but care must be taken that angioplasty/stent does not prevent future surgical procedures.

- If an aneurysm is present, it should be addressed at the time of revascularization or should not jeopardize a future repair.

- If there is significant disease in the common femoral artery, surgical bypass is recommended.

- If both iliac and common femoral artery disease is present, a hybrid approach of femoral endarterectomy and iliac revascularization should be performed.

- Surgical bypass/endarterectomy is recommended if for some reason the blockage(s) cannot be fixed by angioplasty/stent, angioplasty/stent has failed previously or if there is combined blockages with aneurysmal disease.

> **Recommendations for Femoro-Popliteal Disease Revascularization**
> - Angioplasty/stent is recommended over surgical bypass for less severe localized blockages (e.g. Type A lesion; page 79) of the superficial femoral artery not involving femoral bifurcation.
> - If the blockage is < 5 cm, in the superficial femoral artery that have poor technical results from angioplasty, stenting should be considered.
> - If the blockage is 5-15 cm in the superficial femoral artery, use of angioplasty with self-expanding nitinol stents (ask your doctor about these) are recommended.
> - If surgical bypass revascularization for femoro-popliteal disease is being considered, it is recommended that additional examination of your veins be done by ultrasound to select a graft candidate.
> - Angioplasty/stent is NOT recommended for blockages below the popliteal artery (below the knee) for intermittent claudication because it is of unproven benefit and potentially harmful. In some circumstances, this may be done for more severe critical limb ischemia disease.
> - Surgical bypass is recommended for diffuse femoro-popliteal disease, blockages < 5 mm, or severe calcification of the superficial femoral artery if risk is low and healthy graft veins are available.
> - The saphenous vein is usually preferred for surgical bypass to the popliteal artery for both above and below the knee. In the absence of a healthy vein graft, a synthetic (e.g. Dacron) bypass can be used below the knee.

Revascularization for Infra-popliteal Disease: The Arteries below the Knee; Anterior and Posterior Tibial

Because the blood flow above the knee is vital to the arteries below the knee, it is imperative that imaging of all vessels be performed prior to any revascularization of the anterior or posterior tibial arteries. Angioplasty is usually not performed below the knee except in cases where a patient has a high risk of amputation and has critical limb ischemia. However, if it is possible to restore blood flow in the arteries above the knee (e.g. femoral and popliteal arteries) in patients with more severe critical limb ischemia, then angioplasty of the anterior and posterior tibial arteries may be considered. It is also possible to perform angioplasty in the arteries above the knee and surgical bypass on the arteries below the knee. Success rates for revascularization below the knee are lower than in above the knee arteries.

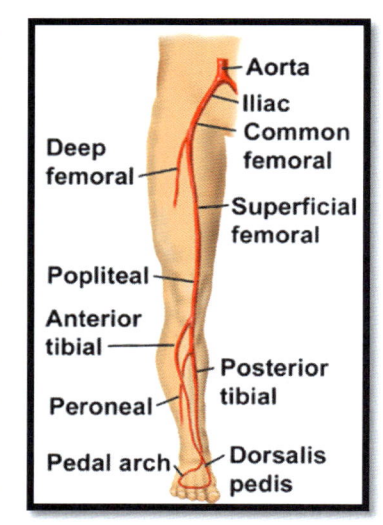

What to Expect When Having Surgical Bypass

Unlike angioplasty where you receive local anesthetic, you will receive general anesthetic when having bypass surgery. This medicine makes you unconscious and you will not feel any pain. In some cases, your doctor may choose to give you an epidural or spinal anesthesia instead. The doctor will inject your spine with medicine to make you numb from your waist down. Your surgeon will make incisions near the blocked artery. Once access is gained to the artery, the surgeon will clamp each end of the blockage and perform the bypass graft. This procedure usually takes 2-4 hours. Following the surgery the medical staff will monitor you in a special area before being cleared to go back to your hospital room. Recovery is longer than with angioplasty, approximately 5-10 days in the hospital and up to 6-8 weeks at home. Your physician will instruct you on wound care and physical activity. It is normal to have leg swelling for an extended period of time. Generally, it is recommended to keep your leg elevated while resting and try to attempt some mild exercise. It is important to make a follow-up appointment with your doctor to make sure the wound has healed, and the surgery was successful. It is very important to call your doctor if:

- You develop a fever
- The wound is red, inflamed or increasingly painful
- You notice abnormal color or cold feeling in your toes
- You have pain at rest similar to walking pain

The table below takes into consideration some advantages and disadvantages of interventions.

Comparison of Angioplasty vs Bypass Surgery

Angioplasty Advantages	Angioplasty Disadvantages
<ul><li>Can be done as an outpatient</li><li>Faster recovery time</li><li>Can be done several times</li><li>Local anesthesia</li><li>Stent can easily be inserted</li></ul>	<ul><li>Lower long term success rates</li><li>Patient may not want multiple interventions</li><li>May have to have bypass anyway</li><li>Higher rates of artery becoming blocked again</li><li>Risk of tear/puncture in artery</li><li>Risk of plaque breaking off into circulation</li></ul>
Bypass Surgery Advantages	**Bypass Surgery Disadvantages**
<ul><li>Long term success rates</li><li>Preferable if more than 2 areas are blocked</li><li>Eliminates need for multiple angioplasties</li></ul>	<ul><li>More potential complications (infection, bleeding, clots, heart attack or stroke)</li><li>General anesthesia used</li><li>Requires taking a vein from another area</li><li>Longer hospital stay</li></ul>

> **The most important thing to remember from this chapter:** An "intervention" is considered an invasive procedure and includes treatment options such as angioplasty/stent or surgical bypass. This should be considered only after conservative treatment has failed to relieve symptoms with medications, reducing risk factors with lifestyle changes first (e.g. stop smoking and start exercising) and risk is low. Patients that need to strongly consider these options include those with leg pain at rest, ulcerations, gangrene or individuals who find the pain during activity is limiting their quality of life at an unacceptable level. Most patients benefit from interventions, however, success rates vary due to the severity and location of the blockage.

References

1) Becker GJ, Katzen BT, Dake MD. Noncoronary angioplasty. Radiology. 1989; 170:921-940.
2) Johnston KW. Iliac arteries: Re-analysis of results of balloon angioplasty. Radiology. 1993; 186:207-212.
3) Norgren L, Hiatt WR, Dormandy JA, Nehler MR, Harris KA, Fowkes FGR;TASC II Working Group. Inter-Society Consensus for the Management of Peripheral Arterial Disease (TASC II). J Vasc Vasc Surg. 2007; 45(S1): S5-S67.
4) Becker GJ, Katzen BT, Dake MD. Noncoronary angioplasty. Radiology. 1989; 170:921-940.
5) Rutheford D and Durham J. Percutaneous balloon angioplasty for arteriosclerosis obliterans: long-term results. In: Yao J, Pearce W, eds, Techniques in Vascular Surgery. Philadelphia, Saunders; 1992: 329-345.

6) Murphy TP, Ariaratnam NS, Carney WI, Marcaccio EJ, Slaiby JM, Soares GM, Kim HM. Aortoiliac insufficiency: long-term experience with stent placement for treatment. Radiology. 2004; 231(1):243-9.
7) Tetteroo E, Van Der Graaf Y, Bosch JL, Van Engelen AD, Hunink MG, Eikelboom BC et al. Randomised comparison of primary stent placement versus primary angioplasty followed by selective stent placement in patients with iliac-artery occlusive disease. Dutch Iliac Stent Trial Study Group. Lancet 1998; 351(9110):1153e1159. 1998; 352:387-353.
8) Klein WM, Van Der Graaf Y, Seegers J, Moll FL, Mali WP. Longterm cardiovascular morbidity, mortality, and reintervention after endovascular treatment in patients with iliac artery disease: The Dutch Iliac Stent Trial Study. Radiology 2004; 232(2):491e498.
9) Bosch JL, Hunink MG. Meta-analysis of the results of percutaneous transluminal angioplasty and stent placement for aortoiliac occlusive disease. Radiology 1997;204(1):87e96.
10) Galaria II, Davies MG. Percutaneous transluminal revascularization for iliac occlusive disease: long-term outcomes in TransAtlantic Inter-Society Consensus A and B lesions. Ann Vasc Surg 2005;19:352-60.
11) Schurmann K, Mahnken A, Meyer J, Haage P, Chalabi K, Peters I. Long-term results 10 years after iliac arterial stent placement. Radiology 2002;224:731-8.
12) Ye W, Liu CW, Ricco JB, Mani K, Zeng R, Jiang J. Early and late outcomes of percutaneous treatment of TransAtlantic Inter-Society Consensus class C and D aorto-iliac lesions. J Vasc Surg 2011;53:1728-37.
13) Indes JE, Pfaff MJ, Farrokhyar F, Brown H, Hashim P, Cheung K. Clinical outcomes of 5358 patients undergoing direct open bypass or endovascular treatment for aortoiliac occlusive disease: a systematic review and meta-analysis. J Endovasc Ther 2013;20: 443-55.
14) Society for Vascular Surgery Lower Extremity Guidelines Writing Group, Conte MS, Pomposelli FB, Clair DG, Geraghty PJ, McKinsey JF, Mills JL, Moneta GL, Murad MH, Powell RJ, Reed AB, Schanzer A, Sidawy AN; Society for Vascular Surgery. Society for Vascular Surgery practice guidelines for atherosclerotic occlusive disease of the lower extremities: management of asymptomatic disease and claudication. J Vasc Surg. 2015;61(3 Suppl):2S-41S.

15) Hirsch AT, Haskal ZJ, Hertzer NR, Bakal CW, Creager MA, Halperin JL, Hiratzka LF, Murphy WR, Olin JW, Puschett JB, Rosenfield KA, Sacks D, Stanley JC, Taylor LM Jr, White CJ, White J, White RA, Antman EM, Smith SC Jr, Adams CD, Anderson JL, Faxon DP, Fuster V, Gibbons RJ, Hunt SA, Jacobs AK, Nishimura R, Ornato JP, Page RL, Riegel B; American Association for Vascular Surgery; Society for Vascular Surgery; Society for Cardiovascular Angiography and Interventions; Society for Vascular Medicine and Biology; Society of Interventional Radiology; ACC/AHA Task Force on Practice Guidelines Writing Committee to Develop Guidelines for the Management of Patients With Peripheral Arterial Disease; American Association of Cardiovascular and Pulmonary Rehabilitation; National Heart, Lung, and Blood Institute; Society for Vascular Nursing; TransAtlantic Inter-Society Consensus; Vascular Disease Foundation. ACC/AHA 2005 Practice Guidelines for the management of patients with peripheral arterial disease (lower extremity, renal, mesenteric, and abdominal aortic): a collaborative report from the American Association for Vascular Surgery/Society for Vascular Surgery, Society for Cardiovascular Angiography and Interventions, Society for Vascular Medicine and Biology, Society of Interventional Radiology, and the ACC/AHA Task Force on Practice Guidelines (Writing Committee to Develop Guidelines for the Management of Patients With Peripheral Arterial Disease): endorsed by the American Association of Cardiovascular and Pulmonary Rehabilitation; National Heart, Lung, and Blood Institute; Society for Vascular Nursing; TransAtlantic Inter-Society Consensus; and Vascular Disease Foundation. Circulation. 2006;113(11):e463-654.
16) Rogers JH, Laird JR. Rogers JH, Laird JR. Circulation. 2007; 116(18):2072-85. Review.
17) Muradin GS, Bosch JL, Stijnen T, Hunink MG. Balloon dilation and stent implantation for treatment of femoropopliteal arterial disease: meta-analysis. Radiology. 2001;221(1):137-45.

18) Hirsch AT, Haskal ZJ, Hertzer NR, Bakal CW, Creager MA, Halperin JL, Hiratzka LF, Murphy WR, Olin JW, Puschett JB, Rosenfield KA, Sacks D, Stanley JC, Taylor LM Jr, White CJ, White J, White RA, Antman EM, Smith SC Jr, Adams CD, Anderson JL, Faxon DP, Fuster V, Gibbons RJ, Halperin JL, Hiratzka LF, Hunt SA, Jacobs AK, Nishimura R, Ornato JP, Page RL, Riegel B; American Association for Vascular Surgery; Society for Vascular Surgery; Society for Cardiovascular Angiography and Interventions; Society for Vascular Medicine and Biology; Society of Interventional Radiology; ACC/AHA Task Force on Practice Guidelines; American Association of Cardiovascular and Pulmonary Rehabilitation; National Heart, Lung, and Blood Institute; Society for Vascular Nursing; TransAtlantic Inter-Society Consensus; Vascular Disease Foundation. ACC/AHA 2005 guidelines for the management of patients with peripheral arterial disease (lower extremity, renal, mesenteric, and abdominal aortic): executive summary a collaborative report from the American Association for Vascular Surgery/Society for Vascular Surgery, Society for Cardiovascular Angiography and Interventions, Society for Vascular Medicine and Biology, Society of Interventional Radiology, and the ACC/AHA Task Force on Practice Guidelines (Writing Committee to Develop Guidelines for the Management of Patients With Peripheral Arterial Disease) endorsed by the American Association of Cardiovascular and Pulmonary Rehabilitation; National Heart, Lung, and Blood Institute; Society for Vascular Nursing; TransAtlantic Inter-Society Consensus; and Vascular Disease Foundation. J Am Coll Cardiol. 2006; 47(6):1239-312.

19) Ansel GM, Silver MJ, Botti CF, Rocha-Singh K, Bates MC, Rosenfield K, Schainfeld RM, Laster SB, Zander C. Functional and clinical outcomes of Nitinol stenting with and without abciximab for complex superficial femoral artery disease: a randomized trial. Catheter Cardiovasc Interv. 2006; 67(2):288-297.

20) Duda SH, Bosiers M, Pusich B, Huttl K, Olivia B, Muller-Hulsbeck S, Bray S, Luz O, Remy C, Hak JB, Beregi JP. Endovascular treatment of peripheral artery disease with expanded PTFE-covered nitinol stents: Interim analysis from a prospective controlled study. Cardiovasc Intervent Radiol. 2002; 25(5):413-418.

21) Gordon IL, Conroy RM, Arefi M, Tobis JM, Stemmer EA, Wilson SE. Three-year outcome of endovascular treatment of superficial femoral artery occlusion. Arch Surg. 2001; 136(2): 221-228.
22) Mewissen MW. Self-expanding nitinol stents in the femoropopliteal segment: technique and mid-term results. Tech Vasc Interv Radiol. 2004; 7(1):2-5.
23) Schillinger M, Sabetti S, Loewe C, Dick P, Amighi J, Mlekusch W, Schlager O, Cejna M, Lammer J, Minar E. Balloon angioplasty versus implantation of Nitinol stents in the superficial femoral artery. NEJM, 2006; 354:1879-1888.
24) Anderson JL, Halperin JL, Albert NM, Bozkurt B, Brindis RG, Curtis LH, DeMets D, Guyton RA, Hochman JS, Kovacs RJ, Ohman EM, Pressler SJ, Sellke FW, Shen WK. Management of patients with peripheral artery disease (compilation of 2005 and 2011 ACCF/AHA guideline recommendations): a report of the American College of Cardiology Foundation/American Heart Association Task Force on Practice Guidelines. Circulation. 2013;127(13):1425-43.

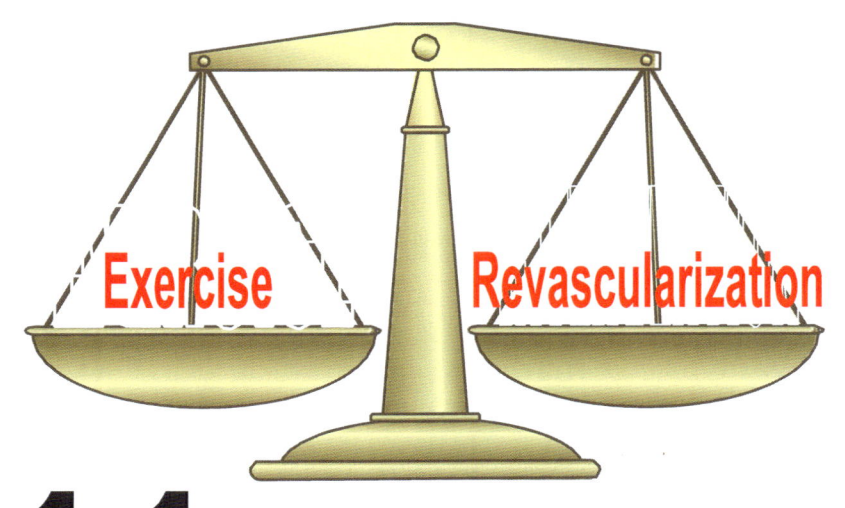

Chapter 11

Exercise or Revascularization: Which is Better for Improving Your Ability to Walk?

In previous chapters we have discussed exercise training and revascularization (angioplasty or bypass surgery) separately. In this chapter we will compare the two treatment options relative to a patient's ability to walk before and after either angioplasty/stent or surgical bypass vs supervised exercise. Keep in mind there are 2 measures of a PAD patient's ability to walk: 1) How long or far one can walk without pain (onset of claudication) and 2) How long or far one can walk in total (peak walking time or distance). Knowing the benefits and expected results of each will make you better informed to choose which is more appropriate for your individual situation. As we have stated earlier, unless your condition has become so severe that you have leg pain at rest, cannot perform activities of daily living without severe claudication or are suffering from ulcers or gangrene, lifestyle changes and medication should be your first course of action.

Evidence that Exercise Improves Walking Ability in Patients with PAD

Supervised exercise has been shown to be one of the best therapies for PAD. **Based on the most recent available evidence, adherence to a**

supervised exercise program is considered the most effective long-term treatment for PAD. Its effectiveness has been demonstrated in over 50 clinical studies and has been shown to be safe and consistently beneficial from the mid-1960's to present. Some of these studies are summarized in the table below. From this table, it is clear that supervised exercise improves both the time (164%) and distance (118%) a PAD patient can walk before the onset of pain starts; and the total time (110%) and distance (97%) a patient with PAD can walk without having to stop. In addition to improved walking ability, studies have also shown increased cardiorespiratory fitness, as measured by aerobic capacity (1,2).

Pain Free Walking and Maximal Walking Before and After Exercise Training in Patients with PAD in Exercise Rehabilitation Studies (meters (m) or time (t) or distance (d)).

Study	Pre-Exercise Pain Free Walking	Post-Exercise Pain Free Walking	Pre- Exercise Total Walking	Post- Exercise Total Walking
Larsen et al., 1966	102 (s)	210 (s)	174 (s)	492 (s)
Alpert et al., 1969	88 (s)	176 (s)	163 (s)	278 (s)
Ericsson et al., 1970	186 (m)	380 (m)	273 (m)	537 (m)
Dahllof et al., 1974	91 (m)	265 (m)	296 (m)	650 (m)
Dahllof et al., 1976	---	170% increase (m)	---	130% increase (m)
Ekroth et al., 1978	108 (m)	392 (m)	283 (m)	720 (m)
Clifford et al., 1980	---	---	299 (m)	535 (m)
Lepantalo et al., 1984	75 (m)	173 (m)	---	---
Rosetzsky et al.,1985	---	---	133 (m)	401 (m)
Ernst et al., 1987	59 (m)	120 (m)	127 (m)	281 (m)
Jonason et al., 1987	114 (m)	197 (m)	430 (m)	717 (m)
Carter et al., 1989	240 (m)	430 (m)	590 (m)	1000 (m)
Mannarino et al., 1991	91 (s)	171 (s)	145 (s)	271 (s)
Feinberg et al., 1992	144 (s)	1218 (s)	306 (s)	2016 (s)
Hiatt et al., 1990	---	---	400 (s)	834 (s)
Hiatt et al., 1994	198 (s)	612 (s)	576 (s)	1038 (s)
Hiatt et al., 1996	156 (s)	360 (s)	558 (s)	906 (s)
Womack et al., 1997	188 (s)	422 (s)	452 (s)	755 (s)
Izquiero et al., 2000	194 (s)	400 (s)	457 (s)	752 (s)
Brendle et al., 2001	271 (s)	525 (s)	623 (s)	890 (s)
Tsai et al., 2002	198 (s)	372 (s)	444 (s)	750 (s)
Gardner et al., 2002	---	189% (m)	---	80% (m)
Gardner et al., 2004	199 (m)	393 (m)	430 (m)	684 (m)
Killewich et al., 2004	190 (s)	413 (s)	443 (s)	752 (s)
Ambrosetti et al., 2004	150 (m)	355 (m)	432 (m)	916 (m)
Gardner et al., 2005	186 (m)	388 (m)	430 (m)	700 (m)
McDermott et al., 2009	158 (s)	332 (s)	461 (s)	696 (s)
Treat-Jacobson et al., 2009	200 (m)	292 (m)	483 (m)	778 (m)
Allen et al., 2010	168 (s)	306 (s)	504 (s)	764 (s)
Murphy et al., 2012	96 (s)	276 (s)	318 (s)	666 (s)
Fokkenrood et al., 2015	210 (m)	390 (m)	373 (m)	555 (m)
Murphy et al., 2015	108 (s)	306 (s)	336 (s)	636 (s)

Supervised exercise is considered by some to be more beneficial than angioplasty [3] for improving the distance PAD patients can walk before getting leg pain and improving the total distance before having to stop and rest. As stated in chapter 8, medications only modestly improve walking distances. Based on this information, **exercise is believed to be more beneficial in improving walking ability than medications!** Several reports have performed a summary of individual studies (like the ones in the above table) called a meta-analysis. The results of these meta-analyses are overwhelmingly in favor of exercise training as a means to improve walking ability in a PAD patient. Improvements in both the onset time of claudication and total exercise show approximately 50%-200% improvements [4,5,6]! A summary of 22 studies reported an improved maximal walking time of 5.12 minutes [7]! Studies that do not show improved walking capacity after exercise training suffer from low patient compliance [8]. Furthermore, home exercise without supervision usually does not work due to low compliance. <u>**Clearly, based on these observations, supervised exercise has the capability to improve a PAD patient's ability to walk. However, exercise training only works if you do it consistently, at least 3 times a week for 30-60 minutes!**</u>

Who is a Candidate for Exercise Training?

Exercise rehabilitation programs are recommended for those patients with early stage PAD (no pain) or with intermittent claudication (pain when you walk, but relieved with rest), or after angioplasty or bypass surgery. In addition, exercise is further recommended for PAD patients because of the increased risk or presence of coronary artery disease to help reduce the risk factors of atherosclerosis (raise your good HDL cholesterol, control blood sugar, reduce blood pressure, reduce body fat, etc.) and prevent heart attacks and strokes. Exercise is very beneficial for those who have diabetes because it can help normalize your blood sugar levels and potentially help you lose weight in combination with a healthy diet. Dedicating yourself to an exercise routine can improve your pain-free walking, slow the progression of the disease and possibly prevent surgery. **Everyone should consult with their doctor on starting an exercise program as soon they are diagnosed with PAD.**

If you have chest pain during exercise you should stop immediately and tell your doctor. However, the leg pain caused by exercise is believed to be beneficial. This uncomfortable feeling, called claudication, is caused by your muscle not getting enough blood and oxygen due to the blocked arteries feeding your legs. Despite being painful, it is not believed to cause damage. In fact, it is believed to be the stimulus for the growth of new blood vessels.

The growth of new blood vessels is the body's natural response to a lack of blood flow to working muscles. For this reason, some believe the best way to improve your walking ability is to walk as long as you can tolerate the pain before having to stop. However, walking for 30 minutes without having to stop is also beneficial.

Evidence that Revascularization Improves Walking Ability in Patients with PAD

Angioplasty. Along with prescription medicine, angioplasty/stent is the most common treatment for intermittent claudication because supervised exercise is not currently paid for by insurance. ***So, the obvious question to ask is, "Will getting an angioplasty/stent improve my walking better than taking my medicine alone?"*** In most cases, an angioplasty/stent will immediately improve a PAD patient's ability to walk who has intermittent claudication. Review of evidence shows a mixture of different arteries, tests and follow-up testing times ranging from 3 months to 2 years. Due to this, it is difficult to directly compare studies, but we will try and summarize the important points and make distinctions between arteries (aorto-iliac vs femoro-popliteal) when possible. One study showed that after 12 months of receiving an angioplasty/stent in the aorto-iliac artery, claudication onset time improved 175% and total walking time improved 160% [9]. Another 12 month study examining angioplasty of the femoro-popliteal artery demonstrated a 52 meter improvement following angioplasty alone in peak walking time and a 20 meter improvement after stenting [10]. In 1-2 year studies that looked at walking performance over 2 years in patients with a combination of aorto-iliac and femoro-popliteal disease, angioplasty/stent improved walking for both onset to claudication and total walking better than medicine alone by 75-200 meters at 3, 6, 12 and 24 months [11,12]. A very recent review reported increases of 44 meters in onset time of claudication and 78 meters in peak walking distant after angioplasty/stent across different time points [13], but up to 500-600 meters in improved walking distances have been reported 6 months after angioplasty/stent [14]. Several studies have demonstrated an early benefit ($\leq$ 1 year) after angioplasty, but not a long-term benefit. Two studies have demonstrated that 2 years following angioplasty a patient's ability to walk was no better than patients who did not receive an angioplasty [15,16]. **Taking all of this into consideration, it is likely that there is a significant improvement immediately after angioplasty/stent lasting up to a year. However, after one year, these gains may start to decline substantially.**

Bypass. We have now shown that patients with intermittent claudication can benefit from angioplasty/stent. _**So, our next question is, "Is surgical bypass any better than angioplasty/stent?"**_ The best evidence to answer this question comes from analyzing all previous studies for both aorto-iliac and femoro-popliteal disease. Although some studies report peak walking time improves by 90% and pain-free walking time by 290% 6 weeks after surgery [17,18], we are unaware of studies that directly compare angioplasty/stent to surgical bypass for changes in walking performance. Other studies do compare complications and how long a blockage remains open between the two revascularization treatments. Due to the more invasiveness of surgical bypass, it is not surprising that it has higher complication rates compared to angioplasty/stent. For aorto-iliac disease, results show surgical bypass has more complications than angioplasty/stent (18.0% vs. 13.4%). However, it is more likely that the area of blockage will remain open after surgical bypass compared to angioplasty/stent at 1 (94.8% vs. 86.0%), 3 (86.0% vs. 80.0%) and 5 years (82.7% vs. 71.4%) [19]. As for comparison in femoro-popliteal disease, similar results have been shown. Angioplasty/stent has fewer complications and result in the blockage remaining open for longer periods of time up to 3 years [20]. From these results, one can conclude that surgical bypass is more durable over 3-5 years compared angioplasty/stent, but also has higher complication rates. As discussed in the previous chapter, there are many reasons why your doctor may favor one revascularization over another. Some patients consider the important factors of pain, hospital stay, and cost into their decisions as well. You should consult with your doctor on what is best for your situation. In general, if your symptoms are severe, lifestyle management has failed and you are not suitable for angioplasty/stent or continue to have pain after several angioplasties/stents, then bypass surgery may be appropriate.

Who is a Candidate for Revascularization?

As you remember from the previous chapter, the two most common revascularization interventions are angioplasty/stent and surgical bypass. As PAD progresses in severity, from no pain to intermittent claudication to pain at rest, these interventions may be required. Fortunately, the prognosis of PAD is generally favorable. The disease progression is slow, with 75% of patients getting better or staying the same and 25% worsening. When considering who should or should not undergo revascularization, general guidelines that indicate a need for intervention are: lifestyle limiting leg pain or pain at rest. Based on these criteria, a candidate for revascularization usually has not improved byoptimal medication and lifestyle management (including exercise training), has pain during daily activities that are limit a desired quality of life/occupation and has too much pain to exercise. Patients may also require revascularization if leg wounds/ulcers are not healing or if a limb is in jeopardy of amputation because tissue is dying. In addition, these patients may have failed one or more previous angioplasties, therefore now requiring surgical bypass.

> **Revascularization Should Be Considered If:**
> - Lifestyle modification (including smoking cessation and exercise) has failed
> - Medication has been maximized and failed
> - Claudication pain exists at rest
> - When there is critical limb ischemia, ulcers, and/or gangrene present
> - Unable to perform daily activities or occupation

Head to Head Comparison of Exercise vs Interventions

In the previous section we demonstrated that most patients who receive an angioplasty/stent can expect significant improvement in walking ability for 1 year. ***So, the next question to ask is, "Is revascularization by either angioplasty/stent or surgical bypass better than supervised exercise training?"*** To date, few studies have directly compared exercise training to revascularization interventions. Two studies done in Oxford, U.K. have suggested that exercise training may be more beneficial than angioplasty for patients with intermittent claudication. The first study [21] (see below; Oxford Study 1) has shown that at 3, 6 and 9 months following angioplasty, which included both aorto-iliac and femoro-popliteal, ABI's were improved (see chapter 2 for ABI) but walking ability was not improved.

> **Angioplasty vs Exercise Training. Oxford Study 1.**
> - 36 claudicants were randomized to angioplasty (n = 20) or 12 months of supervised exercise (n = 16)
> - **Results:**
>   – Angioplasty: Although ABI increased, No benefit in peak walking time or the onset of pain
>   – Supervised exercise improved: Peak walking time improved DESPITE no ABI improvement
>   – Supervised exercise superior to angioplasty for improving functional capacity regardless of ABI changes.
>
> Creasy TS et al. Eur J Vasc Endovasc Surg 1990; 4(2):135-140

However, this study did show that exercise training resulted in better pain-free walking at 6, 9 and 12 months. But no improvement in ABI was detected following exercise training. This may suggest that angioplasty did improve the vessel blockage, but this improvement did not result in increased blood flow to the muscles or improved walking ability. The exercise improved a patient's ability to walk and likely improved muscle without decreasing the blockages in the arteries.

A second Oxford study (*see below; Oxford Study 2*) [3] has supported these findings and concluded that exercise training will improve a patient's ability to walk without pain better than angioplasty. Furthermore, this study showed that patients with femoro-popliteal disease and no aorto-iliac disease improved both onset to claudication and total distance at 6, 9, 12 and 15 months after exercise. However, patients with aorto-iliac disease did not improve their walking ability.

Angioplasty vs Exercise Training. Oxford Study 2.

- 56 Intermittent claudicants (28 had femoro-popliteal disease, 28 had aorto-iliac disease) were randomized to angioplasty or 15 months of supervised exercise training
- Results
  - Angioplasty improved ABI, exercise training did not
  - Exercise training improved distance a patient could walk before claudication started and total distance at 6, 9, 12 and 15 months
  - Angioplasty did not improve walking at any time point
  - Patients with femoro-popliteal disease and no aorto-iliac disease improved both onset to claudication and total distance at 6, 9, 12 and 15 months after exercise
  - However, patients with aorto-iliac disease did not improve their walking ability after exercise
  - Exercise training is superior to angioplasty, but it is possible that patients with femoro-popliteal disease benefit more from exercise training than those with aorto-iliac disease

Perkins JM, et al. Eur J Vasc Endovasc Surg. 1996; 11:409-413.

In a larger, more recent trial on patients with intermittent claudication, it was shown that at 6 months patients who participated in a supervised exercise program were able to improve their ability to walk before pain developed more than those who had angioplasty/stent (899 meters vs 679 meters) [22]. At 12 months, the supervised exercise group also improved more (943 meters vs 806 meters) than the angioplasty/stent patients. In addition to improving the distance before the onset of pain, supervised exercise also improved the total distance a patient could walk before having to stop compared to angioplasty/stent at 6 months (1,138 meters vs 755 meters) and at 12 months (1,034 vs 826 meters). Despite all of these functional measures being better for supervised exercise patients, the investigators did not report these to be statistically different. However, based on these results, the supervised exercise group was able to walk approximately 2 football fields farther than those who had angioplasty/stent. Practically, many patients believe this is significantly better.

The CLEVER Study. Perhaps the best study to date to compare exercise versus angioplasty with a stent placement is the study, "Claudication: Exercise Versus Endoluminal Revascularization (CLEVER) [23,24]. This study directly compared walking ability after 6 and 18 months of either medication only, supervised exercise or angioplasty with stent in patients with blocked aorto-iliac arteries. Six month results showed both supervised exercise and angioplasty with stent improved walking ability more than medication alone. More importantly, at 6 months supervised exercise increased walking times better than angioplasty with stent. At 18 months both exercise and angioplasty improved walking better than medication alone. However, there was no difference between exercise and angioplasty with stent placement.

Another study compared angioplasty, supervised exercise training and the combination of the two in patients with femoro-popliteal disease [25]. Results showed that all three treatments were equally effective in improving walking after 1 year. Considering all of these results, your best first approach to improving intermittent claudication should be exercise training. Supervised exercise training appears to improve walking ability both short-term and long-term.

In support of supervised exercise, other meta-analysis studies (combining results from different studies) have concluded that patients with intermittent claudication may benefit from angioplasty/stent alone for a period of time, but provides no additional benefit over supervised exercise alone [26] and that only supervised exercise had significant value over no treatment [27]. Other comparisons have concluded **angioplasty/stent can improve walking over the short-term of less than 12 months, but supervised exercise is recommended for long-term disease management** [28]. Furthermore, a review of 35 studies including 7,475 patients with intermittent claudication revealed only exercise training improved both maximal walking distance (150 meters) and onset of claudication distance 39 meters) [13]. Few studies have directly compared the utility of surgical reconstruction (bypass surgery) to exercise training. As discussed earlier, **reconstructive bypass surgery does improve blood flow and usually relieves symptoms of leg pain**

immediately, allowing for longer walking distances. One study has shown that the addition of exercise training to bypass surgery further increases walking distances [17], making the combination of the two better than either alone.

The truth in all this data is that if you are experiencing intermittent claudication you should first try to manage all risk factors for atherosclerosis including optimal medication. You also have a choice between supervised exercise and revascularization to improve your claudication. Both will relieve your leg pain. You will likely receive more immediate relief following revascularization vs exercise. But, if you maintain an exercise program it is preferred long-term over revascularization [15]. It is recommended you try a supervised exercise program first because it is safe, less expensive and non-invasive. In many cases this can improve and manage claudication. If lifestyle limiting claudication is not resolved, a revascularization procedure can then be discussed with your doctor. Although surgical interventions are necessary for those PAD patients with advanced disease states, as with all surgery, there are potentially increased risks for complications. Choosing a revascularization procedure depends on the type of lesion and its location. **A combination of these therapies; medication, a healthy lifestyle, revascularization and exercise, is the best strategy. This will give immediate improvement in pain and walking ability for the longest period of time.** This has been supported in studies showing that when angioplasty is added to supervised exercise training the onset to claudication and total walking distance is improved compared to exercise alone at 6 months, 1 year and 2 year in both the aorto-iliac (78% greater at 2 years) and femoro-popliteal (38% greater at 2 years) arteries [29].

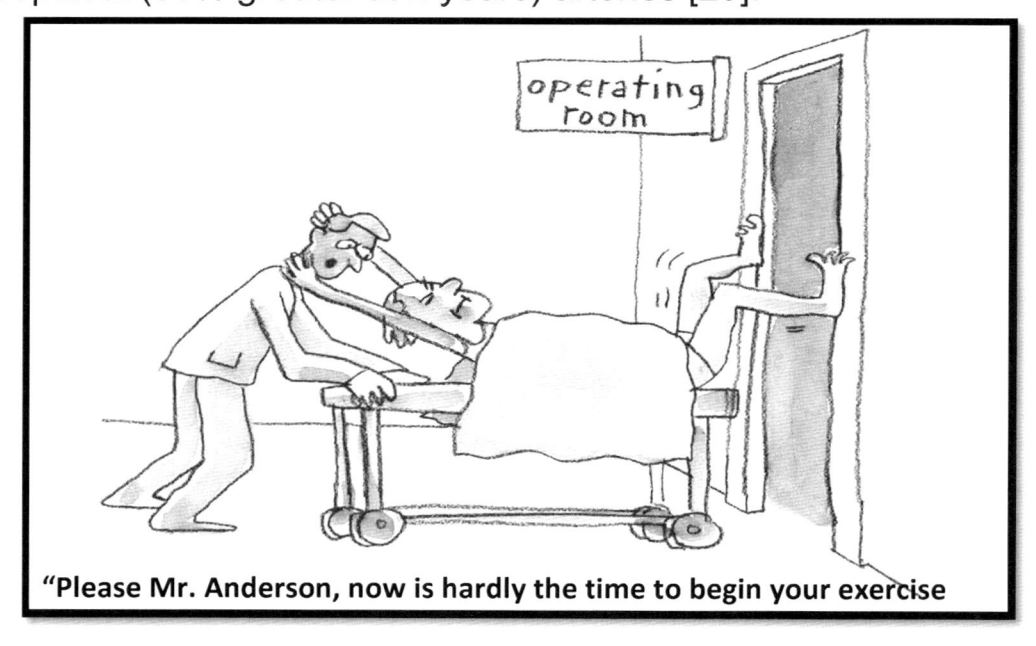

"Please Mr. Anderson, now is hardly the time to begin your exercise

> **The most important thing to remember from this chapter:** Exercise, angioplasty and bypass surgery have all been shown to improve your ability to walk without pain and should be considered complimentary to each other. If possible, supervised exercise should be considered first because of its long-term benefit.

References

1) Duscha BD, Robbins JL, Jones WS, Kraus WE, Lye RJ, Sanders JM, Allen JD, Regensteiner JG, Hiatt WR, Annex BH. Angiogenesis in skeletal muscle precede improvements in peak oxygen uptake in peripheral artery disease patients. Arterioscler Thromb Vasc Biol. 2011; 31(11):2742-8.
2) Parmenter BJ, Dieberg G, Smart NA. Exercise training for management of peripheral arterial disease: a systematic review and meta-analysis. Sports Med. 2015; 45(2):231-44.
3) Perkins JMT, Collin J, Creasy TS, Fletcher EWL, Morris PJ. Exercise training versus angioplasty for stable claudication. Long and medium term results of a prospective, randomised trial. Eur J Vasc and Endovasc Surg. 1996; 11(4):409-413.
4) Gardner AW and Poehlman ET. Exercise rehabilitation programs for the treatment of claudication pain: a meta-analysis. JAMA. 1995; 274(12):975-980.
5) Lane R, Ellis B, Watson L, Leng GC. Exercise for intermittent claudication. Cochrane Database Syst Rev. 2014 Jul 18;7:CD000990.
6) Vemulapalli S, Dolor RJ, Hasselblad V, Schmit K, Banks A, Heidenfelder B, Patel MR, Jones WS. Supervised vs unsupervised exercise for intermittent claudication: A systematic review and meta-analysis. Am Heart J. 2015;169(6):924-937.

7) Watson L, Ellis B, Leng GC. Exercise for intermittent claudication. Cochrane Database Syst Rev. 2008; (4):CD000990.
8) Gelin J, Jivegård L, Taft C, Karlsson J, Sullivan M, Dahllöf AG, Sandström R, Arfvidsson B, Lundholm K. Treatment efficacy of intermittent claudication by surgical intervention, supervised physical exercise training compared to no treatment in unselected randomised patients I: one year results of functional and physiological improvements. Eur J Vasc Endovasc Surg. 2001;22(2):107-13.
9) Murphy TP, Soares GM, Kim HM, Ahn SH, Haas RA. Quality of life and exercise performance after aortoiliac stent placement for claudication. J Vasc Interv Radiol. 2005;16(7):947-53.
10) Krankenberg H1, Schlüter M, Steinkamp HJ, Bürgelin K, Scheinert D, Schulte KL, Minar E, Peeters P, Bosiers M, Tepe G, Reimers B, Mahler F, Tübler T, Zeller T. Nitinol stent implantation versus percutaneous transluminal angioplasty in superficial femoral artery lesions up to 10 cm in length: the femoral artery stenting trial (FAST). Circulation. 2007;116(3):285-92.
11) Nylaende M, Abdelnoor M, Stranden E, Morken B, Sandbaek G, Risum Ø, Jørgensen JJ, Lindahl AK, Arnesen H, Seljeflot I, Kroese AJ. The Oslo balloon angioplasty versus conservative treatment study (OBACT)--the 2-years results of a single centre, prospective, randomised study in patients with intermittent claudication. Eur J Vasc Endovasc Surg. 2007;33(1):3-12.
12) Nordanstig J, Taft C, Hensäter M, Perlander A, Osterberg K, Jivegård L. Improved quality of life after 1 year with an invasive versus a noninvasive treatment strategy in claudicants: one-year results of the Invasive Revascularization or Not in Intermittent Claudication (IRONIC) Trial. Circulation. 2014;130(12):939-47.
13) Vemulapalli S, Dolor RJ, Hasselblad V, Subherwal S, Schmit KM, Heidenfelder BL, Patel MR, Schuyler Jones W. Comparative Effectiveness of Medical Therapy, Supervised Exercise, and Revascularization for Patients With Intermittent Claudication: A Network Meta-analysis. Clin Cardiol. 2015; 38(6):378-386.

14) Hobbs SD, Marshall T, Fegan C, Adam DJ, Bradbury AW. The constitutive procoagulant and hypofibrinolytic state in patients with intermittent claudication due to infrainguinal disease significantly improves with percutaneous transluminal balloon angioplasty. J Vasc Surg. 2006;43(1):40-6.

15) Whyman MR, Fowkes FG, Kerracher EM, Gillespie IN, Lee AJ, Housely E, Ruckley CV. Is intermittent claudication improved by transluminal angioplasty? A randomized control trial. J Vasc Surg. 1997; 26:551-557.

16) Nordanstig J, Gelin J, Hensäter M, Taft C, Österberg K, Jivegård L. Walking performance and health-related quality of life after surgical or endovascular invasive versus non-invasive treatment for intermittent claudication--a prospective randomised trial. Eur J Vasc Endovasc Surg. 2011;42(2):220-7.

17) Lungren F, Dahllhof A, Lundholm K, Schersten T, Volkmann R. Intermittent claudication-surgical reconstruction or physical training? A prospective randomized trial of treatment efficiency. Ann. Surg. 1989; 209:346-355.

18) Regensteiner JG, Hargerten ME, Rutherford RB, Hiatt WR. Functional benefits of peripheral vascular bypass surgery for patients with intermittent claudication. Angiology. 1993; 44:1-10.

19) Indes JE, Pfaff MJ, Farrokhyar F, Brown H, Hashim P, Cheung K. Clinical outcomes of 5358 patients undergoing direct open bypass or endovascular treatment for aortoiliac occlusive disease: a systematic review and meta-analysis. J Endovasc Ther 2013;20: 443-55.

20) Antoniou GA, Chalmers N, Georgiadis GS, Lazarides MK, Antoniou SA, Serracino-Inglott F, Smyth JV, Murray D. A meta-analysis of endovascular versus surgical reconstruction of femoropopliteal arterial disease. J Vasc Surg. 2013;57(1):242-53.

21) Creasy TS, McMillain PJ, Fletcher EW, Collin J, Morris PJ. Is percutaneous transluminal angioplasty better than exercise for claudication? Preliminary results from a prospective randomized trial. Eur J Vasc Surg. 1990; 4(2):135-140.

22) Spronk S, Bosch JL, den Hoed PT, Veen HF, Pattynama PM, Hunink MG. Intermittent claudication: clinical effectiveness of endovascular revascularization versus supervised hospital-based exercise training-randomized controlled trial. Radiology. 2009;250(2):586-95.

23) Murphy TP, Cutlip DE, Regensteiner JG, Mohler ER, Cohen DJ, Reynolds MR, Massaro JM, Lewis BA, Cerezo J, Oldenburg NC, Thum CC, Goldberg S, Jaff MR, Steffes MW, Comerota AJ, Ehrman J, Treat-Jacobson D, Walsh ME, Collins T, Badenhop DT, Bronas U, Hirsch AT; CLEVER Study Investigators. Supervised exercise versus primary stenting for claudication resulting from aortoiliac peripheral artery disease: six-month outcomes from the claudication: exercise versus endoluminal revascularization (CLEVER) study. Circulation. 2012 Jan; 125(1):130-9.

24) Murphy TP, Cutlip DE, Regensteiner JG, Mohler ER 3rd, Cohen DJ, Reynolds MR, Massaro JM, Lewis BA, Cerezo J, Oldenburg NC, Thum CC, Jaff MR, Comerota AJ, Steffes MW, Abrahamsen IH, Goldberg S, Hirsch AT. Supervised exercise, stent revascularization, or medical therapy for claudication due to aortoiliac peripheral artery disease: the CLEVER study. J Am Coll Cardiol. 2015; 65(10):999-1009.

25) Mazari FA1, Khan JA, Carradice D, Samuel N, Abdul Rahman MN, Gulati S, Lee HL, Mehta TA, McCollum PT, Chetter IC. Randomized clinical trial of percutaneous transluminal angioplasty, supervised exercise and combined treatment for intermittent claudication due to femoropopliteal arterial disease. Br J Surg. 2012; 99(1):39-48.

26) Ahimastos AA, Pappas EP, Buttner PG, Walker PJ, Kingwell BA, Golledge J. A meta-analysis of the outcome of endovascular and noninvasive therapies in the treatment of intermittent claudication. J Vasc Surg. 2011;54(5):1511-21.

27) Kruidenier LM, Viechtbauer W, Nicolaï SP, Büller H, Prins MH, Teijink JA. Treatment for intermittent claudication and the effects on walking distance and quality of life. Vascular. 2012;20(1):20-35.

28) Liu J, Wu Y, Li W Wang S. Endovascular treatment for intermittent claudication in patients with peripheral artery disease: A systemic Review. Ann Vasc Surg. 2014; 977-982.

29) Greenhalgh RM, Belch JJ, Brown LC, Gaines PA, Gao L, Reise JA, Thompson SG; Mimic Trial Participants. The adjuvant benefit of angioplasty in patients with mild to moderate intermittent claudication (MIMIC) managed by supervised exercise, smoking cessation advice and best medical therapy: results from two randomised trials for stenotic femoropopliteal and aortoiliac arterial disease. Eur J Vasc Endovasc Surg. 2008;36(6):680-8.

References from Table

Larsen OA and Lassen NA. Effect of daily muscular exercise on patients with intermittent claudication. Lancet 1966; 19:1093-1096.

Alpert JS, Larsen A, Lassen NA. Exercise and intermittent claudication: Blood flow in the calf muscle during walking studied by xenon-133 clearance method. Circ. 1969; 39:353-359.

Ericsson B, Haeger K, Lindell SE. Effects of physical training and intermittent claudication. Angiology 1970; 21:188-192.

Dahllof AG, Bjorntorp P, Holm J, Schersten T. Metabolic activity of skeletal muscle in patients with peripheral arterial insufficiency: Effect of physical training. Eur J Clin Invest. 1974; 4:9-15.

Dahllof AG, Holm J, Schersten T, Sivertsson R. Peripheral arterial insufficiency: Effect of physical training on walking tolerance, calf blood flow and blood flow resistance. Scand J Rehab Med. 1976; 8:19-26.

Ekroth L, Dohllof AG, Gundevall B, Holm J, Schersten T. Physical training of patients with intermittent claudication. Surgery 1978; 84:640-643.

Clifford PC, Davies PW, Hayne JA, Baird RN. Intermittent claudication: Is a supervised exercise class worthwhile? BMJ 1980; 281:1503-1505.

Lepantalo M, Sundberg S, Gordin A. The effects of physical training and flunarizine on walking capacity in intermittent claudication. Scand J Rehab Med. 1984; 16:159-162.

Rosetzsky A, Struckmann J, Mathiesen FR. Minimal walking distance following exercise treatment in patients with arterial occlusive disease. Ann Chir Gynaecol. 1985; 74:261-264.

Ernst EEW, Matrai A. Intermittent claudication, exercise and blood rheology. Circulation. 1987; 76:1110-1114. Jonason T and Ringquist I. Effect of training on the post-exercise ankle blood pressure reaction in patients with intermittent claudication. Clin Physiol. 1987; 7:63-69.

Carter SA, Hamel ER, Patterson JM, Snow CJ, Mymin D. Walking ability and ankle systolic pressures. J Vasc Surg. 1989; 10:642-649.

Mannarino E, Pasqualini L, Innocente S, Scricciolo V, Rignanese A, Ciuffetti G. Physical training and antiplatelt treatment in stage II peripheral arterial occlusive disease: Alone or combined? Angiology. 1991; 42:513-521.

Feinberg RL, Gregory RT, Wheeler JR, et al. The ischemic window: A method for the objective quanitation of the training effect in exercise therapy for intermittent claudication. J Vasc Surg. 1992; 16:244-250.

Hiatt WR, Regensteiner JG, Hargarten ME, Wolfel EE, Brass EP. Benefit of exrcise conditioning for patients with peripheral arterial disease. Circulation. 1990; 81(2):602-609.

Hiatt WR, Wolfel EE, Meier RH, Regensteiner JG. Superiority of treadmill walking exercise versus strength training for patients with peripheral arterial disease. Implications for the mechanisms of the training response. Circulation. 1994; 90(4):1866-1874.

Hiatt WR, Regensteiner JG, Wolfel EE, Carry MR, Brass EP. Effect of exercise training on skeletal muscle histology and metabolism in peripheral arterial disease. J Appl Physiol. 1996; 81(2):780-8.

Womack CJ, Sieminski DJ, Katzel LI, Yataco A, Gardner AW. Improved walking economy in patients with peripheral arterial occlusive disease. Med & Sci in Sports & Exer. 1997; 29(10):1286-1290.

Izquierdo-Porrera AM, Gardner AW, Powell CC, Katzel LI. Effects of exercise rehabilitation on cardiovascular risk factors in older patients with peripheral arterial occlusive disease. J Vasc Surg. 2000; 31:670-671.

Brendle DC, Joseph LJO, Corretti MC, Gardner AW, Katzel LI. Effects of exercise rehabilitation on endothelial reactivity in older patients with peripheral arterial disease. Am J Cardiol. 2001; 87:324-329.

Tsai JC, Chan P, Wang CH, Jeng C, HSIEH MH, Kao PH, Chen YJ, Liu JC. The effects of exercise training on walking function and perception of health status in elderly patients with peripheral arterial occlusive disease. J Int Med. 2002; 252:448-455.

Gardner AW, Katzel LI, Sorkin JD, Goldberg AP. Effects of long-term exercise rehabilitation on claudication distances in patients with peripheral arterial disease: A randomized control trial. J Cardio Pulm Rehab. 2002; 22:192-198.

Gardner AW, Killewich LA, Montgomery PS, Katzel LI. Response to exercise rehabilitation in smoking and nonsmoking patients with intermittent claudication. J Vasc Surg. 2004; 39(3):531-538.

Killewich LA, Macko RF, Montgomery PS, Wiley LA, Gardner AW. Exercise training enhances endogenous fibrinolysis in peripheral arterial disease. J Vasc Surg. 2004; 40:741-745.

Ambrosetti M, Salerno M, Boni S, Daniele G, Tramarin R, Pedretti RF. Economic evaluation of a short-course intensive rehabilitation program in patients with intermittent claudication. Int Angiol. 2004; 23(2):108-113.

Gardner AW, Montgomery PS, Flinn WR, Katzel LI. The effect of exercise intensity on the response to exercise rehabilitation in patients with intermittent claudication. J Vasc Surg. 2005; 42:702-709.

McDermott MM, Ades P, Guralnik JM, Dyer A, Ferrucci L, Liu K, Nelson M, Lloyd-Jones D, Van Horn L, Garside D, Kibbe M, Domanchuk K, Stein JH, Liao Y, Tao H, Green D, Pearce WH, Schneider JR, McPherson D, Laing ST, McCarthy WJ, Shroff A, Criqui MH. Treadmill exercise and resistance training in patients with peripheral arterial disease with and without intermittent claudication: a randomized controlled trial. JAMA. 2009; 301(2):165-74.

Treat-Jacobson D, Bronas UG, Leon AS. Efficacy of arm-ergometry versus treadmill exercise training to improve walking distance in patients with claudication. Vasc Med. 2009; 14(3):203-13.

Allen JD, Stabler T, Kenjale A, Ham KL, Robbins JL, Duscha BD, Dobrosielski DA, Annex BH. Plasma nitrite flux predicts exercise performance in peripheral arterial disease after 3months of exercise training. Free Radic Biol Med. 2010; 49(6):1138-44.

Murphy TP, Cutlip DE, Regensteiner JG, Mohler ER, Cohen DJ, Reynolds MR, Massaro JM, Lewis BA, Cerezo J, Oldenburg NC, Thum CC, Goldberg S, Jaff MR, Steffes MW, Comerota AJ, Ehrman J, Treat-Jacobson D, Walsh ME, Collins T, Badenhop DT, Bronas U, Hirsch AT; CLEVER Study Investigators. Supervised exercise versus primary stenting for claudication resulting from aortoiliac peripheral artery disease: six-month outcomes from the claudication: exercise versus endoluminal revascularization (CLEVER) study. Circulation. 2012 Jan; 125(1):130-9.

Fokkenrood HJ, Lauret GJ, Verhofstad N, Bendermacher BL, Scheltinga MR, Teijink JA. The effect of supervised exercise therapy on physical activity and ambulatory activities in patients with intermittent claudication. Eur J Vasc Endovasc Surg. 2015; 49(2):184-91.

Murphy TP, Cutlip DE, Regensteiner JG, Mohler ER 3rd, Cohen DJ, Reynolds MR, Massaro JM, Lewis BA, Cerezo J, Oldenburg NC, Thum CC, Jaff MR, Comerota AJ, Steffes MW, Abrahamsen IH, Goldberg S, Hirsch AT. Supervised exercise, stent revascularization, or medical therapy for claudication due to aortoiliac peripheral artery disease: the CLEVER study. J Am Coll Cardiol. 2015; 65(10):999-1009.

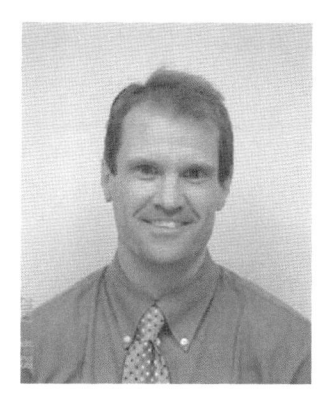

Brian Duscha is an Exercise Physiologist at Duke University Medical Center and has been studying cardiovascular disease for over 20 years. His research includes cardiopulmonary exercise testing, rehabilitation and studying clinical outcomes of patients with peripheral artery disease (PAD), heart failure (HF), coronary artery disease (CAD) and type 2 diabetes mellitus (T2DM). His interest is in prevention, specifically exercise training as a secondary prevention tool in disease populations and exercise amount and intensity in at risk populations. His primary focus in PAD is on the use of exercise to increase small blood vessel growth, skeletal muscle metabolism, comparing exercise to angioplasty and the use of home-based mobile technologies to reduce risk factors. He has coordinated several large National Institutes of Health funded clinical trials on how exercise training improves cardiovascular populations and has over 50 scientific publications in the field.